# THE VERBAL ABUSE RECOVERY WORKBOOK

# The Verbal Abuse Recovery Workbook

## Healing from Emotional Abuse

Christine E. Murray, LCMHC, LMFT

**R**

ROCKRIDGE
PRESS

Interior and Cover Designer: Mando Daniel
Art Producer: Sara Feinstein
Editor: Brian Sweeting
Production Manager: Jose Olivera
Production Editor: Melissa Edeburn

Illustration used under license from iStock.com.

Paperback ISBN: 978-1-64876-773-9 | eBook ISBN: 978-1-63807-462-5
R0

# CONTENTS

This workbook belongs to:

_____

# INTRODUCTION

Congratulations on taking an important step forward in your healing journey by picking up this workbook. Admitting your life has been impacted by verbal abuse and beginning to take active steps to heal are no easy feats. In fact, these steps to start your recovery are some of the most difficult ones to take. It's hard to admit how much another person's words and actions have hurt you and then to reach out for help.

I hope the *Verbal Abuse Recovery Workbook* will become an important tool for you to use in your healing journey. In my nearly two decades of work in the mental health and domestic violence fields, I've seen how deeply verbal abuse can affect people's lives, relationships, and mental well-being. Countless counseling clients, research participants, and people I've met through my advocacy work have shared with me their stories of verbal and other forms of abuse, and these stories have helped me understand how complex verbal abuse can be.

In addition to my professional experiences, I've also personally experienced verbal abuse within the context of a romantic relationship. I've been on my own journey of recovery from abuse, and I've learned some valuable (if sometimes painful) life lessons from that experience that I'll share throughout this workbook.

Verbal abuse can be defined as a pattern of using hurtful words and related actions to gain and maintain power and control over another person. Verbal abuse can occur in all types of relationships—romantic relationships, friendships, relationships with family members, and those in the workplace. Some people face verbal abuse in just one relationship, whereas others experience verbal abuse in multiple relationships at different points in their lives. This workbook is designed to be helpful no matter which category you fall into.

It's normal to have a lot of difficult emotions in the aftermath of verbal abuse, and this is expected. You may feel anxious, confused, frustrated, and even ashamed of or embarrassed about your experiences. Some people's emotions grow further into a traumatic response and may result in mental health symptoms such as depression, anxiety disorders, and posttraumatic stress disorder (PTSD). For this reason, along with the value that professional support can add to the verbal abuse recovery process, it's important to seek the help of a trained mental health professional if you're concerned about the severity of any symptoms you're facing. This is especially important if your symptoms are affecting your work, relationships, and motivation, or causing you a lot of distress. At the end of this book, you'll find a list of resources to help you find a professional in your area.

There should be no shame in acknowledging that you've faced verbal abuse. Abuse can happen to virtually anyone, despite the stereotype that abuse is typically experienced by people who are weak, vulnerable, or from certain demographic backgrounds. Throughout this book, I'll use the term *victim* to refer to someone who is currently facing abuse and the term *survivor* to refer to someone whose experiences are in the past. This book is mostly written for survivors of past verbal abuse, although many people start their recovery journey while they're still facing abuse. I hope this workbook will offer support, whether you have experienced verbal abuse recently or in the distant past.

Healing from verbal abuse takes time. Sometimes it happens in leaps and bounds, and other times, it feels like small but meaningful steps forward. Be patient with yourself as you move through the recovery process. This workbook is designed to offer information, exercises, and strategies that you can use to move forward during this process. I recommend that you work through this workbook from start to finish, but please give yourself permission to use it in the way that is most helpful to you. Toward the end of the book, you'll find a glossary with definitions of some key terms that are discussed throughout the chapters. These terms appear in bold.

If you've experienced verbal abuse, you've been through a painful experience that is likely impacting your life in different ways. Recovering from verbal abuse isn't an easy process, but it can help you find ways to transform those hurtful experiences into opportunities to discover new personal strengths. Remind yourself to keep taking small steps forward, and one day, you'll be amazed at how far you've come. My hope is that this workbook will be a valuable tool along the way.

# PART I

# AN INTRODUCTION TO VERBAL ABUSE

In part 1 of this workbook, we'll cover important background information about verbal abuse to set the stage for the later chapters on the recovery process. Chapter 1 provides an overview of the dynamics of verbal abuse, including common signs and consequences of verbal abuse. Chapter 2 focuses on understanding some of the behavior patterns and motivations of people who perpetrate verbal abuse. Learning more about these aspects of verbal abuse can help you better understand your experiences and how they have affected you. As you read these chapters, keep these important points in mind: The abuse you experienced was *not* your fault. The abuser was fully responsible for their words and actions. And, although the abuse was painful, you *can* heal from those experiences and grow stronger in the process.

# CHAPTER 1

# WHAT IS VERBAL ABUSE?

When you buy a new appliance or piece of technology, what comes first in the accompanying instruction manual? Almost always, it's a basic description of the item, such as where to find the on/off switch and what all the other buttons and features are called. It's helpful to start with the basics, whether we're talking about appliances, technological items, or the process of recovering from verbal abuse. In our case, we'll start this workbook by gaining a basic understanding of the dynamics of verbal abuse, and then we'll cover some other features, such as signs of abuse and common consequences for victims and survivors. To get started, I'll share a bit of my own story.

## Recovery Story: My Own Experiences with Verbal Abuse

When I was in an abusive relationship, I didn't realize right away that I was experiencing verbal abuse. My abuser didn't usually say outright mean things like, "You're stupid," "You're ugly," or "You're worthless." Instead, the verbal abuse was a lot more subtle and was combined with other forms of abuse. I knew how much his words and actions were hurting me, but it was hard for me to describe my feelings and experiences because they didn't match up with the way I understood verbal abuse at the time. I didn't generally hear from him the specific words that I viewed as abusive, so it didn't compute that I was facing abuse until I had the chance to read a textbook on the topic and learned that verbal abuse is about more than just mean words.

*Note: All the other stories in this book are hypothetical examples and are not based on any individual person.*

## THE DEFINITION OF VERBAL ABUSE

Let's revisit the definition of verbal abuse that I shared in the introduction to this workbook: **Verbal abuse** can be defined as a pattern of using hurtful words and related actions to gain and maintain power and control over another person. Sometimes verbal abuse *does* involve blatant mean words like *stupid, ugly,* and *worthless.* However, verbal abuse also can involve more subtle words and actions, such as speaking in a disparaging tone, trying to confuse or manipulate another person, and withholding kind, positive words.

A one-time or isolated use of mean words or a hurtful tone is not necessarily an indicator of an abusive relationship. Most of us have moments of anger or conflict when we say things we regret later. We all make mistakes at times and say or do things we wish we could take back. The difference between healthy and abusive dynamics in relationships is that healthy relationships involve people acknowledging and taking responsibility for their hurtful words and actions and taking steps to make positive changes; in abusive relationships, an abusive person typically does not genuinely accept responsibility or make real efforts to change their behaviors.

## COMMON SIGNS OF VERBAL ABUSE

Because hurtful words and behaviors can happen even in healthy relationships, it can be difficult to determine when verbal abuse is happening. One of the most common signs of abuse—verbal and otherwise—is that the person who is perpetuating the abuse is trying to gain or maintain power or control over the other person. Abusers use abusive words and behaviors because they're trying to make themselves appear more powerful and make the other person or people appear weaker or under their control.

Another common aspect of verbal abuse is a tendency for the abuser to blame the victim or otherwise deny accountability for their actions and how they are impacting the other person. So, the abuser may say things like, "I only said that because you did something to upset me," "You deserve this," or "You're too sensitive and are overreacting." Someone who is facing verbal abuse often feels like they're in the middle of a mind game. Identifying verbal abuse involves looking at an overall pattern of words, behaviors, and responses of the perpetrator.

# Five Warning Signs of Verbal Abuse

Five warning signs of verbal abuse are:

1. The abuser says hurtful words and withholds positive words.

2. The victim feels confused and hurt by the abuser's words and actions, even if they can't always quite put their finger on why.

3. There is a pattern of hurtful words and actions, not just isolated or one-time incidents.

4. The abuser blames the victim for the abuser's own actions.

5. The abuser fails to take accountability for their words and actions.

## HOW DOES VERBAL ABUSE SHOW UP IN DIFFERENT RELATIONSHIPS?

Verbal abuse can happen in all kinds of relationships. You may have experienced verbal abuse from a romantic partner, a parent, a child, another family member, a friend, a coworker, a boss, a teacher or coach, a neighbor, or a fellow member of a community group or spiritual/religious community. In any of these relationships, verbal abuse can occur on its own or alongside other types of abuse, such as physical, sexual, emotional, and/or financial abuse.

Verbal abuse occurs in all directions in relationships, involving, for example, people with the same or different gender identities and people with different or similar levels of power within their social system (e.g., between same-level colleagues or a boss and employee in a work setting). Sometimes there is just one abuser and one victim, but situations with more than one abuser and/or victim are possible. For example, on a sports team, a group of players might gang up on another group of players, such as if a group of seniors verbally abuse and harass a group of freshmen on a high school team. The nature of the relationship in which verbal abuse occurs can impact the dynamics and consequences of the abuse, so let's look at a few examples how verbal abuse can play out in different types of relationships.

### FAMILY

Verbal abuse that occurs within families can be especially painful, given how close family relationships often are and how much time people often spend with their family members. Children who grow up with verbally abusive parents may think such hurtful words and experiences are normal. Because of the high level of influence parents have on their children's lives, children often internalize the negative messages they hear from their parents. So, for example, if a child hears that they'll never amount to anything, they may start to believe this about themselves. And children—especially adolescent or adult children—can verbally abuse their parents, and verbal abuse between siblings and from extended family members can occur as well.

### FRIENDS

A friendship, as compared with relationships with family members, is usually a more voluntary type of relationship, so it may seem as though it would be easier to end a friendship with someone who verbally abuses you. However, people often are quite emotionally attached within their friendships, making this type of verbal abuse especially painful. Because of the important social support that close friendships provide, ending a friendship because of verbal abuse can be a very isolating experience.

### ROMANTIC RELATIONSHIPS

*Intimate partner violence* refers to abuse that happens between current or former partners in a romantic relationship. Although people often associate domestic violence with physical abuse, verbal abuse is a common occurrence within abusive intimate relationships. Abusive partners may use hurtful words to demean their partners and make them feel as though they don't have other options than the abusive partner. Although domestic violence is a crime in most jurisdictions, verbal abuse on its own is often not illegal unless it involves communicating threats of physical harm. As a result, victims of verbal abuse may face barriers to accessing supportive resources (e.g., a protective order) in their community.

### AT WORK

People should be able to conduct their work in a physically and emotionally safe environment. However, a verbally abusive boss or coworker can create a hostile, toxic climate at work. This can hinder an employee's ability to do their job and advance in their career. And because people gain income through their work, it may be difficult for a victim of workplace verbal abuse to leave the toxic work setting. They also may be reluctant to report their abuser's actions because they fear losing their job or facing retribution.

## HOW DOES VERBAL ABUSE MAKE YOU FEEL?

As a child, you probably heard the saying, "Sticks and stones may break my bones, but words can never hurt me." This saying has a nice ring to it, but there's not a lot of truth to it. In reality, hurtful words and actions *can* hurt you. Pushing aside feelings such as sadness, anger, or disappointment from hurtful words doesn't mean those feelings aren't real and won't have an impact on you.

If you were taught from an early age to ignore hurt feelings, you may find a lot of unresolved emotions buried beneath the surface. Ignoring feelings usually doesn't make them go away. Instead, unprocessed feelings tend to build up and come out in unhelpful ways. Acknowledging that those feelings are there is an important first step in your recovery process. In this section, we'll explore some of the common feelings that people who have been verbally abused may experience.

### ANXIOUS

Anxious feelings are understandable in uncertain situations. A verbally abusive relationship is uncertain because you never know when the abuser will hurt you. Most people aren't abusive all the time, and they may even be kind and supportive sometimes. Many people who have faced verbal abuse say they feel like they're "walking on eggshells" around their abuser, in that they're not sure what might incite their abuser to rage. It makes sense that feelings of anxiety and nervousness can linger long after the abusive relationship is over.

### CONFUSED

For people who have faced verbal abuse, confusion can have many sources. It's normal to feel confusion when you're questioning your experiences with verbal abuse: Why is this person treating me this way? Is there something wrong with me? How can I get the abuse to stop? Will this person continue to hurt me even if I end my relationship with them?

In addition, abusers may intentionally use tactics to confuse and manipulate their victims, such as by gaslighting them (we'll talk more about gaslighting in chapter 2). If your experiences with verbal abuse have left you feeling confused, know that you're not alone. Sorting through your confusing thoughts and emotions will be an important part of the healing process.

### ASHAMED

The verbal abuse you experienced was not your fault. You don't have to carry any shame or embarrassment about the abuse. However, many victims and survivors of abuse *do* feel very ashamed of their experiences. You might be embarrassed to tell other people what you've been through, making you reluctant to reach out for help. You might feel as though you've let yourself down or disappointed people who are important to you. We'll discuss how to work through these feelings later in this book. For now, try to remind yourself that any shame associated with the abuse should rest with the abuser, not with you.

### LOW SELF-ESTEEM AND SELF-DOUBT

When you have faced a relationship (or more than one relationship) in which someone has intentionally disparaged you and put you down, a natural emotional response is to have negative feelings toward yourself, such as low self-esteem and self-doubt. This is especially true if you continue to ruminate over your abuser's hurtful words toward you. Recovering from verbal abuse involves working through these hurts and building your sense of self-worth and ability to trust yourself.

### PTSD

**Posttraumatic stress disorder (PTSD)** is a diagnosable mental health disorder that involves a specific set of emotional and cognitive responses to a traumatic event or series of events. Features of PTSD include anxiety, hypervigilance, avoidance of reminders of the traumatic event, and reexperiencing the event, such as through flashbacks or nightmares. Mental health disorders, including PTSD, can only be diagnosed by a qualified mental health professional. If you're concerned that you may be experiencing symptoms, turn to the Resources section toward the end of this book to find information on connecting with professional help.

### OTHER EMOTIONS

Every survivor's experience of verbal abuse is unique, and so are their emotional responses. Acknowledge and honor any emotions that you're facing, in addition to the emotions listed earlier. These may include sadness, anger, resentment, and fear, as well as any other emotions that make sense to you. Be mindful of how your emotions may come in waves over time throughout your recovery process. You may feel relieved and at peace one moment, and then, moments later, you might feel sad, anxious, or angry. Later in the book, we'll discuss ways to work through these feelings. Grant yourself permission to feel any emotions that arise—there's no right or wrong set of emotions that come up as a result of having been verbally abused.

## WITHOUT HEALING, VERBAL ABUSE CAN AFFECT YOU IN THE LONG TERM

Without an intentional approach to healing, you run the risk of becoming bitter or stuck in the past, even as more time comes between you and your experiences of abuse. Unhealed trauma can have negative impacts on people's long-term mental health, relationships, and even career success and financial well-being. That said, be patient as you move forward toward recovery and healing, because it can take a long time. You don't have to be fully healed to have a fulfilling life. Every step you take along the healing journey will bring new opportunities for growth.

When you've faced verbal abuse, it's important to be intentional about healing from those experiences. Some healing can come naturally as time passes, but time alone won't necessarily resolve all the effects of abuse on your life. Being intentional about healing from verbal abuse—such as by working through the content and exercises in this workbook and by seeking professional support—can help you move in a more positive direction toward the healthy life, mindset, and relationships you desire.

# Self-Assessment:
# Your Experience with Verbal Abuse

Reflect on your experiences of having been verbally abused by rating how much you agree with each of the following statements on a scale from 1 to 10 (1 = *completely disagree*; 10 = *completely agree*). Once you have completed your self-assessment, reflect on your answers and how they can inform your goals and intentions in using this workbook.

\_\_\_ I consider the verbal abuse that I faced to be a traumatic experience.

\_\_\_ My experiences with verbal abuse currently impact my mental health.

\_\_\_ My experiences with verbal abuse currently impact one or more relationships in my life.

\_\_\_ Sometimes I feel overwhelmed by my emotions related to my experiences with verbal abuse.

\_\_\_ I have upsetting memories related to the verbal abuse.

\_\_\_ My sense of self-worth was impacted by my experiences of verbal abuse.

\_\_\_ I am committed to being intentional about my healing and recovery from verbal abuse.

## THIS BOOK WILL HELP YOU FIND WAYS TO HEAL

In this chapter, we've covered some of the basics to help you understand the dynamics of verbal abuse and how it plays out in different types of relationships. We've also explored how verbal abuse can impact victims' and survivors' lives in many ways, including their emotional and mental health. This background information has established the importance of being intentional about the journey of healing from verbal abuse.

The rest of this workbook will provide you with more information and tools to help you take steps forward in your healing journey. In the next chapter, we'll explore some of your abuser's patterns and behaviors that may have been especially distressing to you. Building on the foundation of the first two chapters, the interactive chapters that follow include tools and exercises to help you work through different aspects of the healing process.

I encourage you to take time to go through each section of the book to gain deeper levels of understanding throughout your abuse recovery process. Keep in mind that your healing journey is yours to create as you go along. The journey may be difficult and painful at times, but trust that you're resolving the hurts of your past and building a brighter future for yourself.

# CONCLUSION

I hope this chapter has helped you understand your own experiences with verbal abuse and to realize that you're not alone. Far too many people have faced verbal abuse, either on its own or combined with other types of abuse, in relationships of all kinds. Recognizing common patterns and dynamics of verbal abuse can help you feel less alone and less ashamed of your experiences.

Verbal abuse has many possible short- and long-term consequences, and you may face some painful emotions and self-doubts. You may be left with many unanswered questions about why the abuser treated you the way they did. You may never know exactly why they did it, but learning more about the patterns and motives of abusers can help you release the self-blame or shame that you feel. Continue to chapter 2, where we'll start to unmask some of the motives and patterns of abusers so you can understand your experiences further.

# CHAPTER 2

# UNMASKING THE VERBAL ABUSER

Throughout your verbal abuse recovery journey, I invite you to really commit to focusing on you—what you need, how you feel, and your vision for your future. Chances are, you've already spent countless hours thinking about the person or people who verbally abused you. You likely tried to figure out what their motivations were, if and how you could ask or influence them to change their words and behaviors, or what in their underlying psychological makeup compelled them to act in such a way.

These types of thoughts make perfect sense—you were trying to make sense of your experiences and promote your safety and well-being in a harmful situation. However, healing and recovery are about *you* and your own growth, and that's the focus of the rest of this book. Before we turn to that focus, in this chapter, we'll address some common patterns that abusive people display.

Our goal here is not to show you how to try to change them—that is likely an impossible task unless they truly want to change on their own. Instead, we'll spend time unmasking common abuse tactics to underscore one important message that is very important for you to keep in mind throughout your healing journey: Your abuser's behaviors weren't really about you after all—they were about choices *they* made, for which *they* are fully responsible. As we discussed in chapter 1, it's understandable if you feel ashamed of your experiences with abuse. However, in reality, any shame or embarrassment associated with verbal abuse should lie with the person who perpetrated it, and not with you as a victim or survivor.

# Recovery Story: Realizing You Are Not Alone

Consider Ashley's story. Ashley is a 28-year-old single woman who grew up with a verbally and emotionally abusive mother. Ashley has been in counseling for anxiety, and her counselor suggested that she join a support group for survivors of abuse. Before joining the support group, Ashley felt very alone and isolated in her experiences because she didn't know anyone else whose parents treated them like her mom treated her. But when Ashley started listening to the stories of the other members of the support group, she couldn't believe how similar their experiences were to her own. Although their stories brought up new questions for Ashley about how people who are abusive learn to act in such similar and hurtful ways, it was empowering for her to learn that she wasn't alone and that her mother's abusive actions were more common than she realized.

## TYPES OF VERBAL ABUSE TACTICS

Abusers can use many different verbal abuse tactics. Verbal abuse can look very different in one situation or relationship versus another, making it especially complicated to identify. Sometimes verbal abuse is easy to spot, but other times, it's much more subtle and difficult to detect, even if it has been going on for a very long time. For these reasons, it's helpful to avoid narrow definitions of verbal abuse. Remember that abusers can be very sneaky and morbidly creative in the words and associated behaviors they use to hurt others.

In this section, we'll explore some common verbal abuse tactics. Consider these as examples of what verbal abuse *may* look like, but remember that your own experiences with verbal abuse might look different from these patterns. A key question to ask yourself as you consider whether a person's words and actions represent verbal abuse is *What is the apparent motive behind this person's words and behaviors?* If it seems as though they're using these tactics to try to control you or hold power over you, that's a key sign that abuse may be present. Even if the other person's actions don't line up exactly with one of the types of verbal abuse listed next, be alert for other possible signs of abuse, and always take steps to promote your physical and emotional well-being.

### NAME-CALLING

**Name-calling** is probably the easiest form of verbal abuse to identify. Name-calling occurs when an abuser uses hurtful words toward the victim, such as by calling them dumb or cursing at them. Beyond these more obvious examples, however, name-calling can be more subtle, such as using nicknames or pet names that they know will hurt you but that others may not immediately recognize as offensive.

## CRITICISM

When a verbal abuser criticizes you, they're making a general statement about something they claim is wrong with you. They may try to minimize the hurt they've inflicted, such as by saying they're "just trying to help," or they're "trying to make you a better person." However, a verbal abuser criticizes with the intent to harm, not to help.

## WITHHOLDING

In some cases, verbal abuse is more about what someone *doesn't* say than what they say out loud. **Withholding** refers to the absence of the level and type of positive words and associated behaviors that could reasonably be expected based on the nature of the relationship. Of course, there are no clear-cut rules for how much affection, positive words, or encouragement are required for any given relationship. However, withholding represents a significant deficit of positive verbal support. Sometimes this is a consistent pattern from the start of a relationship, whereas in other cases, a person will use verbal withholding after a period of more consistent interactions. Withholding is complicated because some people are naturally more or less verbally affectionate and positive than others. The key here is that the abuser does the withholding intentionally and with the intent to harm.

## THREATENING

**Threatening** words and behaviors can be part of an overall pattern of verbal abuse. Threats may include physical harm but also other potentially hurtful actions such as threatening harm to one's emotions, career or finances, parenting situation, or status or reputation. In addition to verbal statements, threats may be accompanied by threatening behaviors, such as speaking aggressively, loudly, or with hostile facial expressions. By using threats, the abuser is typically attempting to intimidate the victim into submission.

## GASLIGHTING

If I said to you, "You did not just read about threatening words and behaviors in the previous paragraph," that would be an example of my attempt to gaslight you. **Gaslighting** happens when an abuser plays mind games to try and confuse the victim or make them question their own reality, perceptions, and sanity. Abusers gaslight when they act in certain ways and then try to deny that a situation happened or convince you that it happened differently than it did. Gaslighting is a particularly difficult type of verbal abuse to experience because it can lead you to question or doubt yourself; over time, this can contribute to deeper feelings of self-doubt and a lack of trust in oneself.

### EXPLOITING VULNERABILITIES

In healthy relationships of all kinds, people can safely be vulnerable and share personal details about themselves, such as their insecurities and potentially embarrassing past experiences. However, abusers can exploit these vulnerabilities in their verbal abuse tactics by bringing them up in hurtful or spiteful ways. For example, if an abuser knows that their victim has insecurities about their confidence at work or school, they may make statements to reinforce those insecurities in an attempt to make the victim feel even worse about themselves.

### PUBLIC EMBARRASSMENT

Verbal abuse often occurs in private, one-on-one settings, but some abusers bring their verbal abuse into the public sphere. This can involve the abuser using any of the abuse tactics mentioned earlier in a public setting, such as calling someone names in front of their friends, family, or work colleagues. Being verbally abused in front of other people can be an understandably shame-filled experience. However, verbal abusers also can use public embarrassment in subtler ways, such as by sharing secret or private information or making a hurtful "joke" at the expense of the other person.

### TECHNOLOGY-FACILITATED VERBAL ABUSE

In today's technology-saturated world, abusers have many technology-based platforms at their disposal. Abusers may use verbally abusive tactics through social media, text messaging, email, apps, and other devices and channels that grant them access to their victims. Virtually any of the types of verbal abuse we've discussed so far could be carried out using a technology-based platform. The ever-present nature of technology in most people's lives makes this form of verbal abuse especially complicated, in that verbal abusers can exploit technology to gain even greater access to their victims than they could through only in-person interactions.

## VERBAL ABUSE AS A TACTIC TO REINFORCE OTHER FORMS OF ABUSE

Verbal abuse can stand alone within a relationship, but it also typically occurs alongside other forms of abuse, such as physical, sexual, or financial abuse. Verbal abuse usually accompanies, and overlaps with, emotional and psychological abuse. Some experts consider verbal, emotional, and psychological abuse to all fall within the same category of abuse that focuses on hurting people through their thoughts and feelings. Abusers may use the hurtful words and behaviors associated with verbal abuse to reinforce the power and control they're trying to maintain over their victims using any and all other forms of abuse. Therefore, if you've faced verbal abuse, it's possible—and perhaps even likely—that you've also faced at least one other form of abuse. Although the primary focus of this workbook is on verbal abuse, many of the same principles we'll discuss can apply to healing from other forms of abuse as well. However, it is important to be intentional about taking steps toward healing and recovery from all the abusive experiences you've faced, so consider additional steps that may help you if the abuse you faced is multifaceted. For example, you may want to join a support group, read books on other forms of abuse, and seek professional help.

## WHEN DOES IT BECOME ABUSE?

It's normal for people who've experienced verbal abuse to question whether their experiences were abusive. Everybody is human and says hurtful things at times. Most of us try to assume the best regarding the people we care about. So, if someone has said or done something hurtful toward us, we may question whether they really meant it or if it's a red flag for more toxic or abusive patterns. How can you tell if hurtful words or behaviors have crossed a line into abusive territory? Some telltale signs include the following:

- The hurtful words or actions aren't just one-time or isolated incidents. There's a pattern of hurtful behaviors over time.
- There is an underlying dynamic of power and control issues at play. The person is using their hurtful words and actions to try to maintain control over you.
- The offender doesn't seem to regret their actions. Even if they offer an apology, they may quickly revert to using similar behaviors. They don't appear to be working to change their behaviors.
- The person who hurt you doesn't accept personal responsibility for their actions. They may even place blame on you.

## The Difference between Healthy Disagreements and Verbal Abuse

In a healthy disagreement, both people are invested in working through their differences, even if they disagree. However, with verbal abuse, one person is intentionally trying to hurt or diminish the other person's feelings and sense of self-worth. Sometimes, even in a healthy disagreement, people say or do things that are hurtful. However, in healthy disagreements, people regret those words or actions and commit to working on themselves so they won't repeat the same patterns. With verbal abuse, the abuser may claim that they're sorry for what they said or did, but they rarely follow through with efforts to make positive changes.

Conflict is a part of all relationships—even healthy ones. It's natural for people to have differences of opinion, and in fact, it's healthy to honor each other's differences within relationships. In healthy relationships, people make space for those differences and work to understand each other's perspectives, even if they don't agree with one another. However, in abusive relationships, an abuser rarely values and honors the opinions, unique thoughts, and feelings of their victim.

### THE GOALS OF VERBAL ABUSE

*Why is this person acting this way?* If you've wondered that about the person who verbally abused you, you're not alone. If you're a person who believes in treating others with kindness and respect, you may assume that others have the same beliefs and feel very confused as to how an abusive person can act and talk the way they do.

Of course, every person is unique and has their own motivations behind their words and actions. In many cases, you can never really know why your abuser hurt you. However, it can be helpful to realize that abusers often try to achieve certain goals through their abusive behaviors—even if you can't fully know their inner motivations. In this section, we'll explore some of those common goals. Consider how well these goals seem relevant to your own experiences with verbal abuse, especially if it helps you understand your thoughts, feelings, and responses related to the abuse.

## POWER AND CONTROL

All abuse occurs within the context of power and control dynamics; the abuser uses the abuse tactics in an effort to gain or maintain power and control over their victim. This is true for verbal abuse, in that the abuser is using the abusive words and associated behaviors to make themselves feel more powerful and dominant within the relationship.

## MANIPULATE

**Manipulation** is a type of mind game in which someone tries to trick or deceive someone else into doing something they want them to do or into getting them to take their side in a disagreement or debate. People who use manipulative behaviors as part of overall patterns of verbal abuse may recognize that they can't influence you in a positive way, so they resort to deception in hopes of tricking you instead.

## BOOST SELF-ESTEEM

When someone uses hurtful words to belittle or dominate you, it's natural to feel like you are the lesser person and that perhaps they see or know things you're missing. However, the vast majority of abusers act the way they do because they don't like themselves or are battling deep-seated insecurities. You may have heard the phrase, "Hurt people hurt people." People who abuse others are often hurting inside or have been hurt by others in the past. Keep in mind, however, that this is no excuse for abuse. Every person faces some hurts and insecurities in their life, and it is the responsibility of each person to learn to process their emotions in healthy ways that don't hurt others.

## CREATE CONFUSION AND DOUBT

Because abusers are driven to maintain power and control, they inherently seem to understand that they need to diminish their victims' sense of clarity and trust in themselves. Therefore, verbal abuse tactics can be used to create confusion and doubt in the minds of victims. This is especially true if abusers alternate between hurtful words and behaviors and positive, affirming ones, which is very common in verbally abusive relationships of all kinds. Very rarely is an abuser hurtful 100 percent of the time. They may have moments of kindness, but even seemingly kind words and actions are often part of the overall manipulation patterns to try to control their victims.

# Five Simple Self-Care Tips

Coping with the hurts and emotions of past or current verbal abuse is not easy, especially with respect to how cruel verbal abusers can be. It's important to practice self-care throughout your recovery journey so you can process your thoughts and emotions in a healthy way. Here are five simple self-care strategies that can be especially helpful for survivors of abuse:

1. **Journal:** Writing down your thoughts and feelings in a journal can help you gain new insights and release your emotions.

2. **Take a walk:** Spending time outdoors exercising offers benefits for both your physical and mental health.

3. **Spend time with a trusted friend or family member:** Prioritize making time for loved ones who help you feel safe and supported.

4. **Listen to uplifting music:** Create playlists or find streaming music stations that help you feel motivated and positive. Enjoy listening as you go about your day.

5. **Give yourself grace:** Release yourself from the expectation that you have to be perfect. View mistakes as opportunities for growth.

## YOU MAY BE ABLE TO RELATE TO SOME OR ALL OF THIS INFORMATION

Every abusive relationship is unique. As we've explored common verbal abuse tactics and the motivations behind them in this chapter, you may have felt as though your experiences matched every word—or you may have thought that some unique aspects of your experiences weren't fully captured.

Know that abuse often doesn't fit neatly into textbook definitions and descriptions; I know this from my firsthand experience. When I was in my abusive relationship, it took me a very long time to recognize it as abusive because what I was experiencing didn't fit neatly into the images of abuse that I had in my mind. However, once I learned more about how the overall power and control patterns within abusive relationships can play out differently, I could see more clearly how my abuser's words and actions throughout the relationship were part of his overall patterns of abuse and manipulation.

As you move forward throughout your verbal abuse recovery journey, honor your own unique experiences, even if they seem different from those of others.

## ACKNOWLEDGE YOUR EXPERIENCE

Being the target of an abusive person is not easy. If you've lived through verbal abuse or any other forms of abuse, it makes perfect sense that those experiences have left you feeling hurt, confused, and anxious. In many ways, as we've seen throughout this chapter, your abuser's goal all along was to leave you hurt, confused, and anxious. This is especially true if your abuser was someone who should have been in a position to be caring and kind to you, such as a parent, romantic partner, friend, or mentor at work.

Give yourself permission to acknowledge that you've been through a very difficult life experience because of the abuse you faced. If you faced only verbal abuse and were never physically harmed, it may be tempting to minimize the extent of your hurts by saying, "Other people have had it worse." And although it may be true that others' lives have been more difficult than yours, it's also true that your own unique experiences with abuse were hurtful to you—and your healing is important, too.

### EVERY SURVIVOR OF VERBAL ABUSE HAS A DIFFERENT STORY

Every survivor of abuse has a unique and important story to tell—and you get to decide whether and how to tell it. You may choose to keep your story to yourself, or you may choose to share it with others. Your choices about sharing your story might change at different points along your healing journey.

As you move forward in the abuse recovery process, keep in mind that you're in the middle of a story about your life and experiences with abuse that is still being written. While you were being abused, your abuser probably told you a lot of hurtful and untrue stories about yourself. However, now that you're in the process of healing and recovering, it's your turn to write your own stories and correct the ones that your abuser wrote about you. You can keep writing your story until it has the ending that you want to create for yourself!

# A Mindfulness Exercise for Difficult Times

Practicing mindfulness can be a helpful way to manage difficult experiences and emotions during the abuse-recovery process. Mindfulness involves bringing your attention to your present state, including your thoughts, feelings, and senses. When you find yourself feeling overwhelmed, consider taking these simple steps to practice mindfulness so you can refocus your attention on the current moment:

- First, set an intention to practice mindfulness in this moment.
- Second, take a few slow, calming breaths until you feel that your mind and body are more at ease.
- Third, notice your surroundings. In your mind, describe three specific things you see near you. For example, you might notice a window in your room, and note that you see green grass, a few trees, and the street in front of the window.
- Fourth, turn your attention to your inner state of being. Complete the following sentences: "Right now, I'm thinking about _____"; "Right now, something I feel in my body is _____"; and "Right now, I feel _____."
- Finally, take a few more slow, calming breaths. If you'd like, set an intention to try to bring more mindfulness to the rest of your experiences throughout the day.

## YOU ARE WORTH HEALING

Verbal abuse can have significant negative effects on survivors' self-esteem. You may question at times whether you *can* heal from the abuse and even whether you're worthy of healing and a better life ahead. Even if you don't fully believe it right now, keep reminding yourself that you're worthy of healing and of a peaceful, fulfilling life. Your mental and emotional well-being matters, and your life does not have to be defined or damaged by the hurt that your abuser caused you.

# CONCLUSION

In the first two chapters of this workbook, we focused on laying a foundation for your healing by covering the basics of the dynamics and common consequences of abuse, and we explored the common tactics that abusers use and motivations that might drive their behaviors. This information can help you better understand your experiences—and know that you're not alone, and the abuse was not your fault.

Now that we have this foundation in place, it's time to move to the next parts of this book. The next several chapters offer interactive opportunities for you to start taking intentional steps toward healing and recovering from verbal abuse. In part 2, we'll focus on the initial stages of recovery, and in part 3, we'll consider how you can stay committed to your healing and well-being over the long term.

# PART II

# THE STAGES OF RECOVERY

Recovering from verbal abuse is a process, not a onetime event. There's no set time for how long the recovery process can take. Everyone's journey toward healing from abuse is unique, although many survivors have some common experiences along that journey. In part 2 of this workbook, we'll cover three common phases of recovery: nurturing yourself through compassion and self-care, acknowledging the verbal abuse, and establishing strong boundaries. Each chapter offers prompts, exercises, and practices to support your healing and recovery. Take your time working through these chapters to get the most out of the resources provided.

# CHAPTER 3

# NURTURE YOUR SELF-COMPASSION, SELF-ESTEEM, AND SELF-LOVE

Enduring verbal abuse, especially over a long period, can tear down victims' and survivors' self-esteem because of the abusers' controlling behaviors, threats, criticism, manipulation, and intimidation. This trauma and the emotional distress of dealing with verbal abuse can leave survivors feeling powerless, confused, overwhelmed, and on edge, and they begin doubting themselves. It's understandable that loving and honoring yourself right now might seem like a foreign concept. However, committing to nurturing yourself through self-compassion and self-love is an essential step toward rebuilding your self-esteem after you've been belittled and berated by your abuser.

Commit to showing yourself kindness, understanding, and forgiveness on your road to recovery. Although it can take time to rebuild your self-esteem after experiencing verbal abuse, you can take intentional steps to build your self-compassion and self-love until it starts to feel more natural. In this chapter, we'll cover useful tools and exercises to help you rebuild your sense of self and honor your whole self—physically, mentally, emotionally, and in relationships with others.

# Recovery Story: Prioritizing Self-Care

After facing verbal abuse, it can be difficult to prioritize caring for yourself. For example, Julia was verbally abused by her father during childhood and experienced an emotionally abusive relationship with her college boyfriend. In both relationships, Julia was told she was worthless, ugly, and stupid. Throughout her healing journey, she has been working to replace these thoughts about herself with more positive beliefs, and she recently began intentionally practicing self-care by taking time to walk, spending time outdoors, and using relaxation strategies.

Despite her best efforts, Julia noticed that she often didn't follow through on her plans to practice these self-care strategies. Sometimes she found herself skipping walks so she could do more work and missing relaxation time to do chores instead. As she reflected on this tendency to pass up opportunities to practice self-care, she realized she felt guilty whenever she started to take time for herself.

Julia noticed that when she began to take steps toward practicing self-care, she felt as though her own needs weren't important. At times, she even heard her father's or former boyfriend's abusive words ring in her ears. Once she realized these patterns, Julia started replacing her guilt-inducing thoughts with more positive, self-supporting beliefs. For example, she reminded herself of the importance of her mental, emotional, and physical well-being. With these more positive beliefs in play, Julia found it easier to prioritize taking time for herself, and she started to stick with her self-care plans more regularly.

## EXERCISE 1: SETTING AN INTENTION FOR HEALING

Some past hurts and trauma can heal naturally over time. However, time offers no guarantees that healing will occur. It's important to be intentional in your approach to your healing journey from past abuse. Without intention, despite time passing, you may continue to bring the old hurts into new situations and relationships. Unresolved past trauma can have long-term impacts on your overall mental and emotional health.

Before delving further into this book, set some meaningful intentions for your healing process. Consider what commitments you're willing to make to support your own abuse recovery journey, and then describe at least one specific step you can take to put this intention into action. Set at least three intentions in the space on page 29.

**Examples:**

*My intention is to commit the time I need to my healing process.*

*The step I will take to put this intention into action is to dedicate at least one hour each week to going through this workbook.*

*My intention is to reach out for help if I feel like I'm in a crisis.*

*The step I will take to put this intention into action is to identify two possible counselors in my community whom I would feel comfortable meeting with.*

It's your turn now.

**1.** My intention is to _____

_____.

*The step I will take to put this intention into action is to* _____

_____.

**2.** My intention is to _____

_____.

*The step I will take to put this intention into action is to* _____

_____.

**3.** My intention is to _____

_____.

*The step I will take to put this intention into action is to* _____

_____.

Many survivors feel as though they lose touch with the person they were before they faced abuse. When you're being abused by someone who is trying to control you, you may lose a sense of who you are and lose sight of certain aspects of your personality, such as your hobbies, your taste in food or music, your ways of thinking, and sources of joy in your life. Some survivors feel that being abused led them to feel less innocent and lighthearted.

In this exercise, take time to reflect on how being abused has affected your sense of connection with yourself. In the space below, reflect on the following questions:

What were you like before you faced verbal abuse?

_____

_____

_____

_____

_____

How did the abuse temporarily change your sense of self or aspects of your personality?

_____

_____

_____

_____

_____

Which aspects of your pre-abuse life do you want to work toward reclaiming during your recovery process?

_____

_____

_____

_____

_____

Your spiritual, existential, and/or religious beliefs can help you find peace, meaning, and support in the aftermath of abuse. What do these areas of life mean to you? If these beliefs are an important part of your life, in what ways—for example, reading books, engaging in spiritual practices, or being in community with others with similar beliefs—can you be more intentional about connecting with them during your abuse recovery process?

_____

_____

_____

_____

_____

_____

_____

_____

_____

_____

_____

_____

_____

_____

_____

_____

_____

_____

_____

_____

_____

_____

As we discussed in the previous exercise, facing verbal abuse can change you and your perspectives on the world around you. Many survivors feel as though they lost parts of themselves as a result of the abuse. The abuse recovery process presents an opportunity for you to re-create yourself into the person you want to become. Now that you're free from the abuse, be intentional about reclaiming the parts of your past self that you want to reclaim and integrating the strength you gained and the lessons you learned through your experiences with verbal abuse. You can emerge from this process as a stronger, wiser version of yourself.

Answer the following questions to help you imagine the person you want to become as you envision your future.

You have survived the trauma of abuse. What new personal strengths and resources have been revealed?

_____

_____

_____

_____

_____

What important life lessons did you learn through your experiences with verbal abuse?

_____

_____

_____

_____

_____

How do you think you can incorporate these personal strengths and life lessons into the person you know you can become as you heal and recover from the abuse?

_____

_____

_____

_____

_____

_____

If you could fast-forward 20 years, how do you hope you will look back on your experiences recovering from abuse? Will you see that they influenced you toward becoming a healthier, stronger person?

_____

_____

_____

_____

_____

_____

Practicing self-care can feel out of reach if we're too idealistic about what practicing self-care actually means. Of course, many of us would love to practice self-care in extravagant ways, like taking a year off work to live at the beach or spending a full week being pampered at the spa. Unless you're one of the very few people who have unlimited time and financial resources, it's important to develop realistic expectations and plans for integrating self-care into your life.

That said, you don't have to totally stop fantasizing about wildly indulgent self-care practices. These fantasies actually can offer you some helpful clues for the types of self-care that would be most meaningful and impactful for you. In this exercise, we'll look for the seeds of possible realities that can be found in your self-care fantasies. Give yourself permission to dream about what your absolutely most wonderful self-care experience would look like, and then identify tiny seeds of realistic strategies that you can pull out of those fantasies.

In the space below, write about what the ultimate self-care experience for you would be. Use as much detail as possible. Where you would be? What you would be doing? Who would be with you? How you would be feeling?

_____

_____

_____

_____

_____

_____

_____

_____

_____

_____

_____

Now have a look at what you wrote about your fantasy self-care experience. What feelings and emotions does this fantasy bring up for you? How would you feel different from how you actually feel today if you could live out this fantasy?

_____

_____

_____

_____

_____

Finally, if you can't make your ultimate self-care fantasy come true in real life, what are some realistic, if smaller, ways you could create some version of those feelings and experiences?

_____

_____

_____

_____

_____

## Start Where You Are Today

You don't have to wait until you feel complete self-love to start treating yourself with love and kindness. Start where you are today, and act with as much self-love and self-compassion as you can find when you're early in the recovery process. As you move further along in your recovery, practicing self-love will likely feel more natural because your inner feelings of self-love and self-compassion will have grown.

Practicing self-care doesn't have to involve a major overhaul of your life. One way to make self-care a more realistic part of your daily life is to focus on making small changes that can ultimately lead to big results. Small positive changes can become healthy habits when you practice them over time. In this exercise, we honor the value of "tweaks" that you can make in different areas of your life to help lead you to greater health and well-being over the long term. In the chart below, identify one small change you could make starting this week in each area of your life. An example is provided for each area to illustrate the types of small changes that can lead to big impacts on your quality of life.

| Area of Your Life | A Small Change I Could Make Starting This Week |
| --- | --- |
| Your physical health | *Example: This week, I could start to go to bed 10 minutes earlier.*<br>This week, I could: _____ |
| Your mental/ emotional health | *Example: This week, I could put aside five minutes a day to pause, focus on my breath, and tune out any noise and stress.*<br>This week, I could: _____ |
| Your finances | *Example: This week, I could bring my lunch one day instead of eating out to save money.*<br>This week, I could: _____ |
| Your work/ career goals | *Example: This week, I could spend 15 minutes organizing my calendar for the next week.*<br>This week, I could: _____ |
| Your relationships | *Example: This week, I could send one text message to tell a friend or family member something I appreciate about them.*<br>This week, I could: _____ |

Note: Once you've identified small steps you can take in each of these areas, draw a star next to the one or two you'd like to put into practice this week.

## PROMPT 2: YOUR POSITIVE QUALITIES

After your abuser has said many hurtful things about you, it can become harder to feel good about yourself. However, you are a valuable person who is worthy of kindness and respect—from others and yourself. Write a list of the characteristics you like about yourself. If you're having a hard time listing your positive qualities, to help you get started, consider asking trusted friends and family members to share what they like about you.

_____

_____

_____

_____

_____

_____

_____

_____

_____

_____

_____

_____

_____

_____

_____

_____

_____

_____

_____

While you're doing the hard work of recovering from past abuse, be sure to nurture and care for yourself along the way. You can show yourself love every day by building opportunities for nurturing and caring for yourself into your daily routine. This treat could be the same every day, such as taking time to drink a cup of your favorite tea and journal, or you could give yourself different small treats each day. Below, list at least 10 small treats that would be meaningful for you. Examples are food or drinks, favorite songs, inspirational quotes, and any other ideas you have for treating yourself as part of your daily routine.

1. _____

2. _____

3. _____

4. _____

5. _____

6. _____

7. _____

8. _____

9. _____

10. _____

## PRACTICE 1: MAKE YOUR SOCIAL MEDIA FEED WORK FOR YOU

If you're not careful, your social media scrolling can lead you to feel worse about yourself, especially if you have a tendency to compare yourself to others. Be intentional about your use of social media to ensure that it's supporting your recovery, not hurting it. Some steps you can take include following accounts and people who inspire you, unfollowing accounts that lead you to negative feelings, keeping the list of people and accounts you follow to a manageable level, and setting time limits for how long you scroll.

Virtually every person struggles with some insecurities in their life. Verbal abusers often exploit their victims' insecurities, so survivors of abuse may face even greater insecurities than people who have not been abused. One way to overcome these insecurities is to work intentionally toward self-acceptance. This involves freeing ourselves from the need to be perfect and affirming that we are worthy, valuable people even though we have weaknesses.

Self-acceptance is more of a process than a destination. Some people eventually arrive at a place of complete self-acceptance, but most of us need to continue to work toward accepting our limitations, insecurities, and perceived weaknesses as we go through different phases of life. In this exercise, consider your journey to self-acceptance by completing the following sentence prompts:

Some of the hardest parts of myself to accept are . . .

_____

_____

_____

The verbal abuse I experienced made it even more difficult to practice self-acceptance because . . .

_____

_____

_____

I can work toward greater self-acceptance by . . .

_____

_____

_____

While I'm working toward greater self-acceptance, I can continue to remind myself that I am . . .

_____

_____

_____

When we set and achieve big or small goals in different areas of life, we experience a sense of accomplishment and a boost of confidence in our abilities. As you're recovering from verbal abuse, you may find it helpful to actively work toward some specific goals that are meaningful for you. For some people, this might mean training for a 5K or a marathon, whereas for others, it may involve saving a certain amount of money or learning a new skill.

It's important to set challenging, yet achievable, goals. Consider a goal you could start working toward that would challenge you to grow, while also giving you a sense of accomplishment along the way. One helpful framework for setting achievable goals is the concept of **SMART goals**: Specific, Measurable, Action-Oriented, Realistic, and Time-Bound. In the space below, map out a plan to work toward a goal that is meaningful for you and that will help build your self-esteem as you continue along your abuse recovery journey.

**Specific:** What specific goal do you want to work toward?

_____

_____

_____

_____

**Measurable:** How will you measure your progress toward this goal?

_____

_____

_____

_____

**Action-Oriented:** What steps will you take to work toward your goal?

_____

_____

_____

_____

**Realistic:** What, if any, adjustments do you need to make to your goal so that it is more realistic and achievable?

_____

_____

_____

_____

**Time-Bound:** What is your ideal timeline for achieving your goal? What are some milestones that will help you track your progress?

_____

_____

_____

_____

## Finding and Creating Inspiration

Be intentional about inspiring yourself. Find and create inspirational quotes, spiritual texts, and any other words of inspiration, and leave reminders of these messages in places where you can easily see them throughout your day. These messages could be placed in your physical space, such as by hanging them on your refrigerator or mirror, and in your virtual space, such as having an inspirational quote as your background image on your computer or phone. Keep these inspirational thoughts in as many places as you can so you have an ever-present sense of focus along your healing journey.

Being verbally abused is a very difficult experience to go through. You have been through a lot, and most likely, you've faced other challenges in life in addition to the verbal abuse. Going through hard times may not be cause for a party (although it might!), but you can take time to find meaningful ways to celebrate your growth and progress. In this exercise, focus on identifying opportunities for celebrating yourself and your growth.

What are you most proud of about surviving verbal abuse? In what areas of your life have you grown stronger as a result of your experiences?

_____

_____

_____

_____

_____

_____

_____

What are some ways you could celebrate yourself for your growth and progress? Would you prefer to celebrate alone or with others? What would your celebration look like?

_____

_____

_____

_____

_____

_____

_____

How have your experiences with abuse impacted your physical health and well-being? If you faced any physical abuse along with the verbal abuse, you may have sustained injuries from your abuser. And even if you didn't face physical abuse, the chronic stress of verbal abuse can affect your health. In the space below, reflect on these effects, along with what you'd like your optimal physical health and wellness to look like at this phase of your life. Then write at least one small step you could take now to begin to make this vision of health a reality.

Forgiveness is an interesting concept. We often think of forgiving others as a relationship dynamic, but forgiveness is much more of an internal process that involves how we work through and release our own pain from the hurts caused by others. As a survivor of abuse, you are empowered to consider what forgiveness means to you and how you want to apply it to your life and experiences. Keep in mind that forgiveness is possible, regardless of whether you ever hear an apology from your abuser.

Some survivors view forgiveness as excusing others for the hurts they caused, so they don't necessarily want to forgive their abusers. For other survivors, forgiveness is more about their own ability to release any bitterness they feel toward their abuser. What does forgiveness mean to you?

_____

_____

_____

_____

How, if at all, would you like to work toward forgiving your abuser and others who have hurt you in the past? In what ways might this help you move forward in your healing process?

_____

_____

_____

_____

## PRACTICE 2: CREATE A HEALING SPACE

The process of abuse recovery can be very difficult at times. One way to support your healing is to create a healing physical space where you feel safe and comfortable. You can use this space to do some of the work of recovery, such as journaling, practicing relaxation and self-care, and reading.

Identify at least one spot in your home that you could designate as a special healing space. This space could be a room, a corner of your couch, or a special chair. Make this space as cozy as possible—for example, you could put a soft blanket there, have tissues on hand for if you need them, and put some sort of inspirational or peaceful quote on display. Create a space—however big or small—where you can feel as relaxed and safe as possible as you move through your recovery process.

As difficult as it can be to forgive others, sometimes the hardest person to forgive is yourself. Survivors of abuse might struggle to forgive themselves for overlooking early signs of abuse, not standing up for themselves, choosing to be in a relationship with their abuser, and other perceived errors in judgment. However, forgiving yourself is important to release feelings of self-blame for the abuse, which was not your fault. In this exercise, reflect on the following questions to begin to work toward forgiving yourself and releasing any blame you feel for the abuse you experienced.

For which aspects of your experiences with abuse are you having a difficult time forgiving yourself?

_____

_____

_____

_____

_____

_____

What steps could you take to begin to work toward self-forgiveness? Examples are seeking counseling, talking about your experiences with a trusted friend or family member, or writing a letter to yourself that reflects self-compassion and forgiveness.

_____

_____

_____

_____

_____

_____

Many people find it easier to care for others than to care for themselves, but you can apply your spirit of nurturing and care for others toward yourself. What are some of the things you do to care for others that you could start to do for yourself as well?

_____

_____

_____

_____

_____

_____

_____

_____

_____

_____

_____

_____

_____

_____

_____

_____

_____

_____

_____

_____

_____

_____

## Recovery Story:
## My Personal Approach to Self-Care

At the start of this book, I shared that I, too, have had personal experiences with verbal abuse in a past relationship. To help illustrate how different self-care practices can be combined to support survivors' progress in the abuse recovery process, I'll share some of my own strategies that were especially helpful early on in my healing journey.

First, I leaned heavily into my support system soon after that relationship ended. This included professional support from a mental health counselor and the support of a few close friends and family members I knew I could call if needed. Second, I committed to a lot of internal work, including learning to recognize and process my emotions, journaling to release my thoughts onto paper, and focusing on nurturing my spiritual life through connecting with my faith community, in addition to doing my own spiritual reading and listening to uplifting music throughout the day. And third, I built some concrete personal goals and plans to work toward and help give me positive experiences to look forward to. This included training to run a race and making some fun plans to travel within the coming year.

These are just some of the ways that I committed to self-care in my personal abuse recovery process. I hope that my story helps you come up with some ideas of how you can combine self-care strategies that are right for you in a way that will offer you the most support and self-nurturing along your healing journey.

# CONCLUSION

After you've faced verbal abuse, it's no easy task to commit to nurturing yourself through self-care, self-compassion, and self-love. Your abuser's words may continue to replay in your mind and lead you to question your worth. However, as we've seen throughout this chapter, committing to self-care and nurturing yourself through the abuse recovery process are important steps. This may feel a bit unnatural at first, but you'll become more comfortable prioritizing your self-care as you gain more practice and see how it helps support your growth and recovery.

# CHAPTER 4

# ACKNOWLEDGE THE VERBAL ABUSE

Being verbally or emotionally abused is a painful, possibly even traumatic, experience. If your heart hurts because of the abuse you faced, know that you're not alone. It's also normal to feel confused or uncertain about your feelings and experiences of verbal abuse. This is especially true if the abuse happened in a relationship with someone you loved or cared for. In this chapter, our focus will be on helping you acknowledge, understand, and process your experiences and emotions—especially the hurtful and painful ones—in the aftermath of the verbal abuse you faced.

## Recovery Story: Recognizing the Impacts of Abuse

Jon recently left what he'd been calling a "toxic workplace" after he finally found a new job. He'd worked at his previous job for five years. About two years into this job, a new manager took over his department, and the culture of his workplace quickly became a cutthroat environment with a constant underlying tone of conflict and competition. The new manager, Susan, especially seemed to have it out for Jon. She frequently belittled his ideas in front of his coworkers and privately ridiculed him, cursed at him, and called him names.

Jon had attempted to report the manager's behavior to Human Resources on two occasions, but each time, he was told that they investigated the situation and found no problems. He decided to keep his head down, focus on his work, and do his job as best he could so he could provide for his family. He'd been searching for a new job for nearly two years when he finally found the right opportunity with a new company.

As Jon got settled into his new job, he began to realize just how deeply his old workplace had impacted him. When he was talking to one of his new coworkers about the toxic culture at his old job and how Susan had treated him, his coworker said, "That doesn't just sound like a toxic culture. That sounds like verbal abuse." At first, the notion of verbal abuse didn't resonate with Jon, but he decided to read more about it so he could

*CONTINUED*

understand what his coworker meant. The more he read, the more Jon realized that Susan *had* been verbally abusing him since she became his manager. Understanding that he had faced verbal abuse and acknowledging the toll it had taken on his mental well-being was an important first step toward Jon's recovery.

Whether you realized that you were facing abuse while it was happening or discovered it later, like Jon did, it's likely that your experiences with abuse have had a lasting effect on you. Acknowledging this effect is one of the most important steps you can take as you begin your verbal abuse recovery process. The activities in this chapter are designed to help you examine and process your experiences to gain self-awareness and insights that you'll continue to develop through other phases of your recovery journey.

## EXERCISE 1: IT WAS WRONG THAT . . .

Abuse of any kind is wrong. There is no place for abusive words or actions in a healthy, supportive relationship. However, because abusers often do not acknowledge the hurt they've inflicted, survivors may need time and support to feel validated regarding the hurt they've faced. In this exercise, practice self-validation by acknowledging that it was wrong that you faced specific incidents of abuse. Begin each statement with the words, "It was wrong that . . . ," and list the ways your abuser(s) wronged you. Repeat this statement as many times as needed for it to be helpful to you.

*Examples:*

- *It was wrong that my boss belittled my work when I had spent so much time and effort on it.*
- *It was wrong that my coworkers stood by and watched while my boss and other coworkers made fun of me.*

It's your turn now:

It was wrong that _____

(*Repeat as often as needed*)

_____

_____

_____

This exercise offers a series of questions to guide you in exploring the power and control dynamics at play in your experiences of verbal abuse. Take time to reflect on each of the questions and write your thoughts in the space provided. Remember that there are no right or wrong answers. Focus on your own experiences, feelings, and observations without judging them.

What were the clues that your abuser was trying to gain and/or maintain power and control over you?

_____

_____

_____

_____

How did your abuser's exertion of power and control impact your thoughts and feelings?

_____

_____

_____

_____

In what ways did your abuser's attempt to gain power over you affect your sense of self-worth?

_____

_____

_____

_____

Looking back now on when the abuse first started to happen, what message do you wish you could tell yourself about how your abuser was trying to hurt and control you through their abusive words and actions?

_____

_____

_____

_____

What is one way you're currently being proactive about regaining your sense of power and control over your own life?

_____

_____

_____

_____

## PROMPT 1: EMOTIONAL BARRIERS

What is getting in the way of your feelings about the verbal abuse you experienced? Write about any thoughts, feelings, messages you received from your abuser, and other barriers (e.g., a busy schedule, tiredness, or lack of alone time) that are currently making it difficult for you to fully experience your emotions related to the verbal abuse you faced.

_____

_____

_____

_____

_____

_____

_____

_____

Abusers often fail to take responsibility for their own words and behaviors, blaming their victims for their abusive actions. In this exercise, we'll explore whether and how victim-blaming played out in your relationship. Write your answers to the questions in the space provided.

What did your abuser say to imply or directly state that you were to blame for their actions?

_____

_____

_____

_____

How did your abuser's actions reinforce their blaming of you? For example, they may have apologized for their actions right afterward but never took any steps to truly try to change their behaviors.

_____

_____

_____

_____

Some victims have experiences with other people (aside from their abuser) that also involve victim-blaming. Who else in your life, if anyone, said or did things to imply that you were to blame for the abuse you experienced?

_____

_____

_____

_____

To what extent did you internalize these victim-blaming messages from others and begin to blame yourself for the abuse? If you had self-blaming thoughts, how did this impact your emotions?

---

---

---

Finally, end this exercise by creating a personally meaningful affirmation that you can repeat to yourself when you have feelings of self-blame or if others say or do things to imply that you were to blame for the abuse. Examples might include: "The abuse was not my fault," or "My abuser is totally responsible for their own actions." In the space below, write the affirmation that will mean the most to you.

---

---

---

It's common for victims and survivors to feel shame for having been abused. This exercise will guide you through an exploration of any feelings of shame or embarrassment you may be carrying in relation to your experiences with abuse. Then we'll walk through a process for releasing shame that you can repeat when these feelings arise.

First, to what extent do you feel shame or embarrassment about your experiences with verbal abuse? What are your fears regarding what other people might think about you if they knew you had faced abuse?

_____

_____

_____

_____

_____

Next, how do feelings of shame or embarrassment impact your life currently? How do they influence how you feel about yourself? How do these feelings impact your relationships, such as your ability to trust others and share your story with them?

_____

_____

_____

_____

_____

1. First, make a statement to acknowledge your feelings. For example, you might say, "I feel shame because I think other people would think I was weak if they knew I'd been treated that way."

   _____

   _____

   _____

2. Second, make an alternative statement to put shame in its rightful place. An example might be, "The only person who should feel ashamed for the abuse I experienced is the person who abused me."

   _____

   _____

   _____

3. Third, develop a plan for reinforcing your commitment to releasing shame. What are some ways you can remind yourself in the future that you don't have to carry shame or embarrassment?

   _____

   _____

   _____

4. Finally, commit to seeking help if your feelings of shame become too much for you to bear on your own. Write at least one professional and one informal support person (e.g., a friend or family member) to whom you could reach out for support if the need arises.

   _____

   _____

   _____

You won't always have the time and attention needed to fully process the thoughts, feelings, and memories connected to your abuse that arise as you go about your days and nights. Memories may come up while you're driving, busy at work, or lying in bed in the middle of the night, trying to sleep.

Even if you can't fully process them in the moment they arise, these transient thoughts, feelings, and memories can offer important clues for your healing process. They might reflect specific areas in which you could take new steps toward further healing.

Keep track of these momentary glimpses into the ongoing inner impact of your abuse so you can revisit them during a better time for healing, such as when you have personal quiet time or when you're meeting with your counselor. Set up a system for recording these thoughts and feelings. You can keep a running note in your smartphone, have an email chain with yourself to write down new ideas, use voice memos to record them, or carry a small notepad with you.

By writing down your thoughts, you can free your mind from the need to keep replaying them. You may feel more at ease knowing that these insights are preserved and can be revisited when you're ready.

## Healing Won't Necessarily Happen on Its Own

One of the key takeaways from this chapter is the importance of bringing intentionality to your verbal abuse recovery process. Being intentional about your healing means that you commit to making the time and space in your life to focus on your recovery.

Every person's needs and experiences for the abuse recovery process are unique, so being intentional starts by considering what will work best for you. This includes the steps you want to take, how much time you can commit to the process, and what type of support you need along the way.

Embrace this opportunity to make the right choices for you. Move forward at a pace that feels safe and comfortable. The key is to bring focus and intentionality to your healing and allow the process to evolve as you move forward in your recovery journey.

You already have a lot of inner strength and resources to help you move forward in your healing journey. However, we all need to develop new knowledge when we're going through hard times we haven't faced before, and that includes the difficult process of recovering from verbal abuse. In this exercise, you'll map out the knowledge you have already, along with what you need or would like to have in terms of additional information to support you in your recovery process.

First, what are some of the key pieces of information you already have about verbal abuse and the abuse recovery process?

_____

_____

_____

_____

_____

Second, what questions do you need answered to help you better understand verbal abuse and the abuse recovery process?

_____

_____

_____

_____

_____

Third, what are some sources of information you could turn to? Take time to search for credible resources—such as books, websites, and workshops—that may be helpful to learn more from, and list them below.

_____

_____

_____

_____

_____

## "The scars from mental cruelty can be as deep and long-lasting as wounds from punches or slaps but are often not as obvious."

—Lundy Bancroft, *Why Does He Do That? Inside the Minds of Angry and Controlling Men*

Write your reflections on this quote. Consider the following questions as a starting point:

What are some of the long-term effects you've faced from verbal abuse?

_____

_____

_____

How does knowing that other people can't see these scars affect you?

_____

_____

_____

What do you wish others knew about the hurts you faced from verbal abuse?

_____

_____

_____

At some point in your healing journey, you may find it helpful to seek out a mental health professional for additional support and guidance. Even if you're not looking for a counselor right now, or if you're already working with one, take the time to think about the characteristics in a professional that you would find helpful. What would make you comfortable working with them? For each characteristic you identify, think of some questions that you might ask a prospective counselor to help you figure out if they're the right person for you. Use the table below to develop your list of characteristics and questions.

| Characteristic | Question(s) I Could Ask |
| --- | --- |
| *Example: Trained in trauma recovery* | *Example: What type of training and experience do you have related to working with clients who are recovering from past abuse?* |

*Note: This exercise could be especially triggering, so be sure to practice self-care as you revisit memories of your abuser's hurtful words toward you. If you don't already have effective self-care practices in place, you may want to skip this exercise for now and revisit it once you have strengthened your coping resources.*

It's likely that you already replay the hurtful words and actions of your abuser in your mind from time to time. For some survivors, there is a constant replay of abuse incidents in their memories. These memories can be distressing, so it's important to learn to process them in an intentional and healthy way. In the spaces provided, reevaluate some of the hurtful things your abuser said or did to you. As you progress through this exercise, remind yourself that you are safe now, that your abuser's hurtful words were not true, and that you deserve to be treated with kindness and respect.

Something your abuser said or did: _____

How deeply did this hurt, on a scale from 1 to 10? (1 = *least hurtful*; 10 = *most hurtful*)

_____

_____

_____

Why did this incident sting so much? What particular vulnerability or insecurity of yours did it target?

_____

_____

_____

_____

What specific emotions did it bring up?

_____

_____

_____

_____

As you look back on that incident, what can you see now that you didn't see then? Focus on how these words or actions were untrue and not reflective of the level of kindness and respect that you deserve.

_____

_____

_____

*Tip: Repeat this exercise five times, and feel free to use the additional space in the back of this workbook to process more incidents.*

### PROMPT 3: IMPACTS IN DIFFERENT AREAS OF LIFE

How are your experiences with verbal abuse impacting your life today? What are the different areas of your life in which you can see lingering effects of the abuse, such as at work, in your relationships, and in your mental and emotional health? How do you think these areas of your life will change as you move forward in your recovery process?

_____

_____

_____

_____

_____

_____

_____

_____

_____

_____

_____

_____

# It's Okay to Admit You've Been Hurt

Depending on how you were raised and the cultural messages you've received from the media, you may have grown up believing it wasn't okay to feel or express certain emotions, such as sadness or anger. Did you hear any of the following messages while you were growing up?

- "Boys don't cry."
- "Don't be sad."
- "Get over it."
- "Just push through it."

Many people grow up feeling as though they have to deny hurt and painful feelings. However, denying feelings doesn't make them go away. In fact, denying your feelings instead of acknowledging and processing them in healthy ways can lead to those feelings building up and coming out in unhealthy ways. Give yourself permission to acknowledge the painful experiences you've faced and your emotional responses to them. Admitting that you've been hurt is often the first step in the process of healing.

### PROMPT 4: PROOF OF YOUR STRENGTH

Consider the following affirmation statement: "I've faced hurtful experiences, but I'm not damaged because of them." Write at least five pieces of evidence that you're a strong person despite your difficult experiences.

1. _____

2. _____

3. _____

4. _____

5. _____

Just because your abuser said hurtful things about you does *not* mean those things are true. You can overcome the lies that your abuser told you about yourself and replace them with more positive, factual beliefs. In this exercise, describe specific lies that your abuser told you or ways that their behaviors led you to have feelings about yourself that you know are not true. Then refute each statement with at least three pieces of evidence to the contrary. Finally, write a more positive, factual statement to replace your abuser's lies.

Lie #1: _____

Evidence to refute this lie:

1. _____

2. _____

3. _____

A more positive, factual statement to replace the abuser's lie:

My abuser said _____,
but the truth is that _____.

*Tip: Repeat this exercise five times, and feel free to use the additional space in the back of this workbook to process even more incidents.*

## PRACTICE 2: RESET BUTTONS

As you process your thoughts, feelings, and experiences with verbal abuse, you'll likely have times when you start to feel emotionally overwhelmed. This may happen in moments when you can't fully work through your thoughts, feelings, and experiences because you need to be present in the moment.

Develop a few emotional reset buttons and practice them so you'll be prepared to navigate these times—for example, if you become anxious about something abuse-related while you're in a meeting at work or dealing with an intense parenting situation with your children.

Some examples of reset buttons are taking a few deep, calming breaths; repeating an empowering statement or mantra (e.g., "It's all going to be okay" or "I can handle this"); or taking a quick time-out in a different room, even if you have to go to the restroom to do so!

These quick reset buttons won't necessarily make all your distress go away, but they can help bring you back into the present moment and calm you down to a point where you can think clearly and act intentionally in the stressful situation you're facing.

Specific incidents of verbal abuse have immediate emotional effects; verbal abuse can also take a long-term emotional toll that may take quite a while to overcome. The long-term emotional effects of abuse often come out in phases over time. You may have moments when you feel elated that you're free from the abuse and other moments when you feel sadness and grief—and sometimes you might just feel exhausted or confused about your feelings.

Create a timeline to depict key moments in your emotional experiences in the time since you faced the abuse. Don't worry about filling in every single thing. Focus on some key events and how you felt about them. Mark the end point on the timeline as today's date, and note any emotions you have today in relation to the abuse you experienced.

*Example:*

| *Fear* | *Rage* | *Relief* | *Empowered* |
|---|---|---|---|
| \| | \| | \| | \| |
| The last abuse incident | The first time I saw my abuser after the abuse ended | My first counseling appointment | Today |

It's your turn now:

| *Fear* | *Rage* | *Relief* | *Empowered* |
|---|---|---|---|
| \| | \| | \| | \| |
| The last abuse incident | | | |

# CONCLUSION

In this chapter, we've examined the nature of the abuse you experienced and the ways that it has impacted your thinking, emotions, and life. Although processing these experiences is undoubtedly painful at times, it can offer new insights and opportunities for healing. You've also built some important skills that you can apply in your ongoing recovery journey, such as learning to process your thoughts and feelings in a healthy way. In the next chapter, we'll move forward into another important skill to support abuse survivors' recovery: the ability to set and maintain healthy, strong boundaries. Read on to learn more and practice skills to help you establish healthy boundaries in different areas of your life.

# CHAPTER 5

# ESTABLISH STRONG BOUNDARIES

Having healthy boundaries helps you keep potentially hurtful people at a distance. In this chapter, we'll explore tools and insights to help you build healthy boundaries in different areas of your life, including your relationships, your schedule, and your commitment to your abuse recovery process.

Healthy boundaries are especially valuable during the recovery process for survivors of abuse. These boundaries can help you manage your interactions with your external environment while also promoting a sense of safety and support internally.

In this chapter, I invite you to consider ways you can build healthy boundaries to protect your physical, mental, emotional, and social well-being. Setting and maintaining these boundaries is a way to prioritize your needs while also fostering healthy relationships with others.

## Recovery Story:
## The Challenges and Benefits of Setting Boundaries

LaTanya is a survivor of verbal and physical abuse by her ex-husband, also the father of her three teenage children. Although LaTanya and her ex-husband have been divorced for more than five years, he continues to try to verbally abuse her and put her down any chance he gets.

Because he has never committed or even threatened physical abuse since their divorce, LaTanya feels that she can't seek legal or law enforcement remedies. However, she is the first person to admit that her ex-husband's ongoing verbal abuse causes her a lot of distress and makes it much more difficult for her to relax and enjoy her time with her children.

Recently, LaTanya started meeting with a mental health counselor. She wanted to learn how to set boundaries with her ex-husband to limit his access to her as much as possible. It hasn't been easy, and in fact, her ex-husband's abuse seemed to escalate once she tried to implement boundaries. However, she's starting to see some clues that the boundaries she's setting are taking effect and helping create more distance from her ex-husband—and a bit more peace within herself.

Wouldn't it be nice if toxic people came with a bright red warning sign? ("Toxic person ahead: Proceed with caution!") Unfortunately, people and relationships don't come with a written warning (unless you happen to know someone who warns you about them). However, you can develop your skills in recognizing signs that it may be wise to keep a distance from another person. Some of these signs: the other person disregards you and your needs, they consistently violate your boundaries, and spending time with them makes you feel worse about yourself.

Take time to reflect on your experiences with people who have had a toxic influence on your life. These experiences likely involved the person or people who verbally abused you, but other toxic people and relationships you've faced in different areas of life may come up as well, such as neighbors, coworkers, or classmates.

Next to the bullet points below, write words that reflect behaviors, feelings, and other warning signs that might signify a toxic person or relationship.

- _____
- _____
- _____
- _____
- _____
- _____
- _____
- _____
- _____

Different types and strengths of boundaries are needed for different kinds of people in your life. Consider the metaphors of a brick wall, a gated fence, and a property line. This approach will help you identify which people (or types of people) you want to have access to you and your life and the level of access you wish to grant them.

Brick wall boundaries are for people whose access to you should be as limited as possible. A gated fence boundary is for those people you want to keep some clear limits around, but you also want to keep an open door to allow for greater access as you get to know them and build trust. With property lines, boundaries are present, but there's enough trust and comfort in the relationship that the boundaries are mutually understood, respected, and not crossed without consent.

In the spaces provided below, list some people you want to set each type of boundary for. You can also include people's characteristics on this list.

Brick wall boundaries:

_____

_____

_____

_____

Gated fence boundaries:

_____

_____

_____

_____

Property line boundaries:

_____

_____

_____

_____

What fears or concerns come up when you think about setting clearer boundaries with others? For example, some people fear that others won't like them if they speak up about a boundary crossing. These fears can get in the way of your ability to set and maintain effective boundaries, so take time to write your thoughts on these fears in the space below.

_____

_____

_____

_____

_____

_____

_____

_____

_____

_____

_____

_____

_____

_____

_____

_____

_____

_____

_____

People often struggle with saying no to invitations, experiences, and requests that other people make of them. However, learning to say no with grace is a skill you can develop, and it can be very valuable in your abuse recovery process. The skill of saying no is also key to having healthy boundaries and to building and maintaining positive relationships with others.

In the space below, write ideas for statements you could use to say no in a kind but firm manner. Although saying no is a complete statement on its own, it's helpful to include a bit of information in the statement that adds kindness to the response. Keep in mind that it's important to avoid offering too much wiggle room—you don't want to give the other person an opening to come back and ask again.

Once you have your list, keep it handy so you can refer to it the next time you're asked to do something you don't want to do.

*Examples:*

*I'm sorry, I don't have the bandwidth to take this on right now.*

*I have to say no this time, but keep me in mind for similar opportunities in the future.*

Just because you set boundaries with others doesn't mean those boundaries will be respected. Sometimes people cross your boundaries unintentionally—maybe they didn't realize that they said or did something that didn't align with a boundary you'd set. Other times, people (especially those who are abusive) intentionally ignore and violate the boundaries you set.

Several factors will impact how you'll want to navigate these boundary violations; these factors include the nature of your relationship with the other person, how safe you feel in the relationship, how receptive you think they'll be to you expressing your concerns to them, and how severe and intentional you view the boundary crossing to be.

This exercise offers questions for you to consider when you're deciding how to respond to a boundary crossing. In the space provided, answer the questions in relation to a recent boundary crossing you faced. You can revisit the questions later on if other boundary crossings arise.

First, how did you know that your boundary had been crossed? For example, what did you observe about the other person's behaviors? What inner signals or feelings did you experience in relation to the boundary crossing?

_____

_____

_____

_____

Second, what steps can you take to process your thoughts and feelings related to this boundary crossing? Consider how to set aside time for reflection, and gain insight into your experiences and emotions before you plan how to respond to the other person.

_____

_____

_____

_____

_____

Third, what are the best options available to address the boundary crossing with the other person? One option may be not addressing it directly with the other person at all, instead focusing on your own healing from any lingering hurt from those experiences.

_____

_____

_____

_____

_____

Finally, from the options identified above, consider the one you think is the best to try. Map out the next steps to take to implement this plan.

_____

_____

_____

_____

_____

## Setting Boundaries Can Be Scary!

It's natural to fear that other people may dislike you if you're more assertive about your boundaries in your relationships with them. As you begin to practice boundary-setting skills, be mindful of any fears or insecurities that arise. Remind yourself that people who value you and honor your relationship will want to understand and honor your boundaries. Seek healthy, affirming relationships with people who respect you enough to honor your boundaries and talk through any differences or disagreements that arise in the process.

Unfortunately, we can't always avoid being in the same place at the same time with people we'd prefer never to see again. If you must be in the same room with your abuser or with someone else you need a very distanced boundary with, it's helpful to have some tools to mentally clear that space in your mind.

A good friend of mine is a therapist who works with college students. She once shared with me a powerful metaphor that she encourages her counseling clients to use when they have to be in the presence of a toxic person. She encourages them to visualize a huge drain on the floor between them and the other person. The drain sucks down any negativity in the space between them.

In the space below, develop a metaphor of a drain, vacuum, or something else you can bring to mind that will help you mentally and emotionally clear the space between you when you must be in the presence of a toxic or hurtful person. Write out details of what you can visualize in these situations to help you bring the image to life when you need it most.

_____

_____

_____

_____

_____

_____

_____

_____

_____

_____

_____

_____

Your experiences with boundaries in your family of origin during childhood can have a significant influence on how you think and feel about boundaries as an adult. How would you describe the boundaries in your family of origin, and how do you think your earliest experiences with boundaries are currently impacting your experiences with boundary setting today?

_____

_____

_____

_____

_____

_____

_____

_____

_____

_____

_____

_____

_____

_____

_____

_____

_____

_____

_____

_____

Boundary setting is a useful skill to apply not just in relationships with others but also in other areas of your life to promote your mental and emotional well-being. These inner boundaries are the focus of the rest of this chapter's exercises.

First, let's consider how barriers can help you protect the space, time, energy, and attention you need to devote to your abuse recovery process. Many barriers and challenges in life can get in the way, including busyness, distractions, procrastination, and feeling overwhelmed by life's demands.

To get started with this exercise, think of possible barriers that could impact your journey of healing from verbal abuse, and list each barrier in the left column of the table. Then, next to each potential barrier you identified, in the right column, write at least one strategy you could use to establish a boundary to protect the time and space you need for your healing process.

| Possible Barriers to My Healing Process | Strategies to Establish Boundaries to Protect My Time, Space, and Energy for My Healing Process |
|---|---|

Rushed decisions can lead you to make choices and commitments that don't honor your boundaries. This is especially true when people ask you to do things that you don't really want to do—particularly if you feel pressured or obligated to say yes.

Practice pausing to give yourself more time before responding to invitations to commitments, events, and other opportunities. Grant yourself permission to take time to think through your decisions so you can process your thoughts and feelings. You may want to practice using specific statements to create opportunities for these pauses. For example, you could say, "Thank you for thinking of me. I'd like to take a few days to think this over, but I promise I'll let you know my decision by the end of the week."

Even if you think you want to say yes to a particular opportunity, pause to create space to reflect before you respond to requests for your time and energy. This practice will help you make the right decision for you, whether you end up saying yes or no.

People often struggle with balancing the demands they face in different areas of their lives, such as work, parenting and family responsibilities, friendships, other relationships, self-care, and hobbies. Keeping all these areas of life in *perfect* balance is an unrealistic expectation, but you can strive for a *manageable* balance in which you feel that your time and attention are aligned with your most important priorities in life.

Having a sense of balance in life is also important for your verbal abuse recovery process—it allows you to preserve the time and energy needed to focus on your healing—and for building an overall long-term quality of life after abuse. In this exercise, take time to reflect on the following questions and write some ideas for fostering a sense of balance in your life.

First, what does the concept of finding balance in your life mean to you?

_____

_____

_____

_____

_____

Second, what are the biggest challenges you face related to finding and maintaining a sense of balance in your life?

_____

_____

_____

_____

_____

Third, what are some specific boundaries that you could put into place to promote balance in the areas of your life that are your highest priorities? For example, you could schedule time for those areas, seek professional coaching, or ask a friend or family member to serve as an accountability partner to help ensure that you're staying committed to your goals for balance in life.

---
---
---
---
---

## PROMPT 3: LEARNING FROM PAST SUCCESSES

You can learn a lot from past successes and challenges with boundary setting. In the space below, dissect one past successful experience and one unsuccessful experience of trying to set or maintain a boundary in your life or relationships. Describe what happened, what you learned, and how you can apply what you learned to future opportunities to set boundaries.

---
---
---
---
---
---
---
---
---

Technology is an integral part of life today, and most of us have nearly constant access to one or more forms of technology. Many valuable technology-based tools are available that can support you on your abuse recovery journey, such as informational websites and online support groups. However, technology can also serve as a barrier to your healing process, such as if it becomes a distraction from the time and attention you need for your healing journey or if you engage with content online that hurts your mood or self-esteem.

Answering the questions below will help you consider boundaries that could be helpful as they relate to your use of technology.

First, on the scale below, which ranges from 0 (*not at all*) to 100 (*completely*), write the word "now" above the line to indicate how much technology is *currently* a distraction or barrier to your healing; focus specifically on how much of your time and attention it takes. Then write the word "goal" to indicate how much *you would like* technology to be part of your life during your abuse recovery process.

0 ⟵——————————————————————⟶ 100

Second, list three to five specific ways that your use of technology could be impairing your abuse recovery process.

1. _____

2. _____

3. _____

4. _____

5. _____

Finally, list three to five steps you could take to set boundaries around your use of technology to foster your emotional and relationship health during your abuse recovery process. For example, you could keep your phone out of reach when you're spending time with friends or family, unfollow social media accounts that leave you feeling worse and replace them with accounts that inspire and motivate you, and disconnect or disable apps or email on your phone at certain times of day (e.g., at bedtime).

1. _____

2. _____

3. _____

4. _____

5. _____

## Healthy Boundaries Are Clear, Yet Flexible

With greater clarity about your needs and expectations about your boundaries, you'll have a better understanding of what steps you may need to take to set and maintain these boundaries in your life and relationships. However, it's also important to maintain some flexibility and adaptability in your boundaries.

Life brings many unexpected changes, and overly rigid boundaries may hinder your ability to respond to different circumstances in your life. For example, let's say you set a boundary that you didn't want your friends, family members, or colleagues to call you after a certain time in the evening so you could focus on your partner and children. However, it's likely that at some point, an emergency or crisis will arise that requires an evening phone call. If your boundary around this is clear, yet flexible, you can be confident that this boundary will generally protect your family time, but you can also respond to exceptional situations.

As you're building healthier boundaries in different areas of your life, leave some wiggle room so you can adapt to the changing circumstances that life will inevitably send your way.

As a survivor of abuse, you have a powerful story that you may want to share with others. This could involve anything from disclosing your experiences of abuse to a new friend to speaking to the media or a large audience at a public awareness event. Many survivors of abuse find it empowering to share their stories with others, although it is certainly not a requirement to heal from past abuse.

Developing boundaries around sharing your story with others is helpful, whether privately or publicly. You can set boundaries related to what parts of your story you share, how and when you share it, and how you might respond if someone reacts to your story in a hurtful way. Answer the following questions to think through the boundaries around sharing your story that might be helpful to you.

First, what are some characteristics that you would want in a person or group of people with whom you may share your story? Examples are good listeners, people who are not judgmental, and those who are trustworthy.

_____

_____

_____

_____

_____

_____

Second, which parts of your story are you most comfortable sharing? Which parts of your story do you want to keep private?

_____

_____

_____

_____

_____

_____

Third, what are some ways you can practice self-care if you feel anxious about sharing your story with others?

_____

_____

_____

_____

_____

_____

_____

Finally, what are some steps you can take if you share your story and the person or people you're sharing it with respond in hurtful, judgmental ways? What boundaries could you put in place even after you've begun to share your story?

_____

_____

_____

_____

_____

_____

_____

PROMPT 4: YOU ARE WORTHY OF HEALTHY BOUNDARIES

Believing that you're worthy of healthy boundaries is an important first step toward building those boundaries. A sense of inferiority or low self-worth can hinder your boundary-setting efforts, especially if other people challenge those boundaries. In the space provided, write a letter to yourself that describes why you are worthy of having healthy, strong relationships in all areas of your life.

_____

_____

_____

_____

_____

_____

_____

_____

_____

_____

_____

_____

_____

_____

_____

_____

_____

_____

_____

_____

People who have faced abuse often want to help others who have had similar experiences. Helping others can give you a sense of purpose and meaning after you've had a traumatic experience. However, listening to others' experiences can also trigger memories and anxiety for survivors. Also, some people may try to take advantage of your willingness to help and ask more of you than you want to provide.

Therefore, if you have opportunities to help others throughout your abuse recovery process, work on establishing boundaries to protect yourself while doing so. The following questions can help you put appropriate boundaries in place to prevent derailing your own healing as you support others. Practice answering them now, using a recent example of when you had a chance to offer some sort of help or assistance to another person.

What are the exciting and positive aspects of this opportunity to help?

_____

_____

_____

_____

_____

_____

_____

What concerns or reservations do you have about this opportunity to help?

_____

_____

_____

_____

_____

_____

_____

_____

What type and level of help can you offer at this time? Consider how much time you can devote to helping others and the specific ways you can offer your help or support.

_____

_____

_____

_____

_____

What signs might alert you that the other person is asking for help that goes beyond what you can offer?

_____

_____

_____

_____

_____

What are specific steps you can take to establish or reinforce your boundaries so you can offer your help but also honor your own needs?

_____

_____

_____

_____

_____

Although this chapter focuses primarily on developing your own boundary-setting skills, it's useful to consider how respecting others' boundaries can help you build healthy boundaries as well. Be intentional about respecting others' boundaries, including both the boundaries they've communicated to you directly and those they've indicated more indirectly, such as in their responses to your actions.

Respecting the boundaries of others gives you practice considering how boundaries are a key part of healthy relationships. Plus, when you're known to be a person who honors others' boundaries, you'll feel a greater sense of integrity when you expect others to do the same.

If you don't have a clear sense of the boundaries that are important to your close friends and family members, consider talking with them about it and asking how you might work together to build positive, healthy boundaries in your relationships with them.

## Recovery Story:
## Be Patient with Learning Boundary Setting

At the start of this chapter, we learned about LaTanya, who was struggling to set and maintain boundaries in her relationship with her abusive ex-husband, especially as they related to her interactions with him around parenting their three teenage children. We learned that LaTanya's ex-husband initially escalated his abusive interactions when she began to set stronger boundaries in that relationship, but eventually she saw some progress.

LaTanya's experience is not uncommon, and many people find that it takes a lot of time and practice to more effectively set and maintain healthy boundaries, as well as respond to boundary violations. Be patient with yourself and others as you work toward building stronger boundaries in your relationships and other areas of your life—especially as you work through other aspects of your abuse recovery process. Take your time as you establish the boundaries you need now to protect the time, space, and energy you need to support your healing.

# CONCLUSION

Virtually everyone who has faced abuse knows the pain and confusion that comes from unhealthy, unsafe boundaries in relationships. Abuse involves the abuser intentionally violating and hurting the well-being of their victim, and healing from these boundary violations is an important part of the overall healing process for survivors.

Learning to set healthy boundaries takes time, practice, and intentionality. Boundary setting is an important skill to build on as you move forward in your journey toward healing from abuse. This skill can also help you in other areas of your recovery process by allowing you to create and protect more opportunities for healing and caring for yourself.

In part 2 of this workbook, we've covered some of the initial stages of the recovery process, from committing to self-care, to acknowledging the hurt you've faced, to building strong boundaries, to protecting your healing. As we move into part 3, we'll take a longer range view toward the ongoing commitment to your healing and recovery. Keep these initial concepts in mind as you move into the long-term work of healing because they will be foundational to your continued progress and growth.

# PART III

# COMMIT TO HEALING

Healing from verbal abuse takes time. Once you're free from the immediate crisis of the abuse, you have an opportunity to begin the long-term journey of healing and recovering. In part 2, we covered some of the earliest phases of abuse recovery, which lay the groundwork for the deeper, ongoing later phases of healing. This includes strengthening your capacity for building safe, healthy relationships with others and beginning to dream about your future.

As we move into part 3 of this workbook, we'll delve into these longer-term abuse recovery processes. All phases of the recovery process can be challenging, but try to keep a positive, hopeful perspective, knowing that these challenges can lead you to a fulfilling life and relationships.

# CHAPTER 6

# LEAN ON YOUR COMMUNITY

Verbal abuse is a relationship-based hurt, so it's understandable if your experiences with abuse have left you struggling to feel safe, trusting, and supported in other relationships in your life. Despite what your abuser may have told you, you are worthy of healthy, kind, and respectful relationships in all areas of your life.

This chapter will help you build trust in relationships, nurture your existing relationships, and build a strong support system. Throughout your abuse recovery process, be intentional about surrounding yourself with people who encourage and uplift you and avoiding those who bring you down and hinder your progress.

## Survivor Story: Overcoming Loneliness

Juan is a 30-year-old sales executive who, by all outward appearances, really has his life together. He lives in a beautiful home, drives a nice car, is well dressed, and is involved in his church and some civic clubs in the community. He has a friendly demeanor and is well liked by neighbors, colleagues, and fellow club members.

Despite these appearances, however, Juan was feeling a deep sense of loneliness. Although he enjoyed being the center of attention at work and club meetings, he admitted that most of his social connections were superficial. He couldn't identify one close friend he could really open up to, and he'd never had a significant romantic relationship.

Juan's feelings of loneliness became almost unbearable, and he decided to seek out counseling for professional help. He was concerned that his loneliness may start spiraling into depression. As his sessions progressed, he and his counselor began exploring how some of Juan's early experiences of bullying and verbal abuse by peers throughout elementary, middle, and high school years led Juan to be leery of trusting others as an adult. He realized that he preferred to keep people at a safe emotional distance because he was afraid of being hurt.

*CONTINUED*

Juan described himself as a "late bloomer." He said that he experienced something of a personal transformation when he went to college in a different state. As the only person from his high school to attend this college, Juan had given himself a makeover before the school year started. He joined a fraternity and felt liked and popular for the first time in his life. However, this time also marked the beginning of his pattern of telling jokes and taking the role of the life of the party to win the approval of others. Since then, he has lived with a constant sense of fear that other people "will find out what's wrong with me."

Juan's counseling process focused on healing his past hurts and learning to build his capacity for healthy relationships with others. He has worked on building relationship skills and learning how to be more open and vulnerable. Although Juan recognizes that the thought of being hurt in relationships is still frightening to him, he is growing in his capacity to trust himself and others and to let others get to know him at a deeper level.

Juan's experiences with relationships following his own verbal abuse may sound very familiar to you. It's completely understandable that you might struggle in relationships when you've been hurt in the past. It may be tempting to close yourself to future relationships (and certainly it's a good idea to maintain as much distance as possible from toxic, hurtful people), but remember that close, supportive relationships are an important part of an overall healthy life. Complete the exercises in this chapter to reflect on your goals for relationships and develop new skills and knowledge that will support high-quality connections in different areas of your life.

For the past several years, my colleagues and I have been working on a community-based initiative to promote healthy relationships. Through that work, we developed a framework for defining a spectrum of quality in relationships of all kinds: the Happy, Healthy, Safe Relationships Continuum (Murray, Ross, and Cannon, 2021). Within this framework, we view safety as the foundation for healthy and happy relationships. In other words, you can't have a healthy or happy relationship if it isn't safe.

**Safe relationships** are free from violence and abuse, and they provide a sense of physical and emotional safety and comfort. In this exercise, complete the following sentence prompts to reflect on what safety in relationships looks like to you.

I feel safe in a relationship when . . .

_____

_____

Some specific actions I see in other people that help me feel safe with them are . . .

_____

_____

My experiences with verbal abuse made me feel unsafe because . . .

_____

_____

Things I can do to care for myself if I feel unsafe in a relationship are . . .

_____

_____

Some of the reasons I deserve to feel safe in relationships include . . .

_____

_____

When you have a physical scar on your skin, the scar tissue is typically more tender and sensitive than the skin around it. Experiencing abuse can leave behind some relational scars in the form of lingering hurts that may be hindering your current relationships.

In the space below, write about any tender spots you still have around relationships as a result of the abuse you faced. Is it difficult for you to trust, like Juan in the case study at the start of this chapter? Do you prefer to keep people at a distance to avoid being hurt? Once you've reflected on any relational scars you have, write about how you'd like to see those scars heal as you move forward in your abuse recovery journey.

_____

_____

_____

### PROMPT 1: RELATIONSHIP EXPECTATIONS

The expectations that we bring into relationships—including our hopes and fears—can impact how we think about and act toward others. Use the space here to write your reflections on your most significant hopes and dreams for relationships, as well as your biggest fears. How do these hopes and fears influence how you approach relationships?

_____

_____

_____

There's a special kind of validation and support you can find in fellow survivors of abuse. People who haven't lived through abuse may find aspects of surviving it difficult to understand. Therefore, a formal support group for survivors can be a valuable resource during your abuse recovery journey. Informal connections with other survivors—such as friends or family members who have gone through similar experiences—can be helpful as well. This exercise will help you research or identify potential connections with other survivors.

First, spend some time searching for information on support groups for survivors of abuse that meet either in person in your local community or virtually online. One tip for finding potential support groups is to focus on the specific type of abuse you experienced or the type of relationship you had with your abuser (e.g., support groups for survivors of intimate partner violence as compared with adult survivors of childhood abuse). If you have a difficult time finding options, consider calling the domestic or family violence agency in your community, or a national hotline, such as the National Domestic Violence Hotline, if you experienced verbal abuse in a romantic relationship. Below, list the options you identified through this search.

Option 1: _____

Option 2: _____

Option 3: _____

Second, search for online communities that may not meet at designated times but that could offer you support or connection with fellow survivors. Many social media accounts have been set up by and for survivors. For example, a colleague of mine and I started the See the Triumph social media campaign (SeeTheTriumph.org, @SeeTheTriumph on Facebook, and @triumphoverabuse on Instagram) based on research we did with survivors of past intimate partner violence. We heard from many survivors who let us know how the messages and information provided through the campaign helped them along their healing journey. Take time to identify potentially helpful online platforms that might help you connect with other survivors via social media, and list the prospects you find below.

Option 1: _____

Option 2: _____

Option 3: _____

Finally, do you have a personal connection with anyone who has shared with you that they have faced abuse? If not, can you think of some well-connected people who might know someone who has had similar experiences to yours? If so, would you feel comfortable asking if they could make an introduction? Below, list any ideas for people you could reach out to.

Person 1: _____

Person 2: _____

Person 3. _____

Once you have developed the previous lists, identify at least one person or group as a starting point for connecting with other survivors at this phase of your recovery process.

### PROMPT 2: SUPPORTING YOURSELF WHEN RELATIONSHIPS ARE HARD

Relationships can be a source of joy, but they can also be a source of hurt, even in healthy relationships. Closer relationships bring the potential for even greater hurts because of how much they mean to us. In healthy relationships, people support each other, work together to talk through these hurts, and develop a stronger relationship as a result. How can you support yourself through relationship hurts so that you can respond to them in a healthy way?

_____

_____

_____

As you think about building a healthy support system to lean into during your abuse recovery process, try thinking like a coach for a sports team. Sports teams are most likely to be successful when teammates bring with them unique strengths and skill sets. For example, a soccer team full of only great goalies would be lacking necessary skills and talents in other positions on the field.

Similarly, an effective support system is likely filled with different kinds of people who can offer different kinds of support. Some may offer emotional support and validation, and others may provide tangible support, such as helping with child care or transportation to counseling appointments. Still other supporters might offer a wealth of information about local community resources.

In the table below, first list the types of support you anticipate would be helpful during your abuse recovery process. Then, next to each, list people who might be able to offer you each type of support. If you have a difficult time identifying people who could offer certain types of support, consider how you might build additional connections to expand your support team.

| Type of Support That Could Help My Abuse Recovery Process | Names of People I Know Who Might Be Able to Provide This Support |
| --- | --- |

# Embrace (Healthy) Conflict in Relationships

It's understandable if you have anxieties and fears around conflict in relationships after you have experienced verbal abuse. Your experiences with conflict with your abuser were likely hurtful, toxic, and unsafe. However, healthy approaches to conflict management are a good thing in relationships! Healthy conflict allows people to work through their differences, learn to understand one another better, and work toward solutions that can strengthen their relationships. As you build healthier relationships, work toward overcoming fears of conflict and embrace the value that healthy conflict management skills can add.

## EXERCISE 5: WHAT YOU NEED TO BE ABLE TO TRUST

Did you know that it can be healthy to be skeptical about trusting new people in your life right away? It can take time to learn whether someone is worthy of your trust. Answer the questions below to reflect on your need in relationships to build trust.

What are some important characteristics that you look for in someone you can trust?

_____

_____

_____

What are some signs that you should be wary of trusting someone?

_____

_____

_____

What are some strategies you can use in relationships to build trust over time? Taking time to get to know someone before sharing your full story with them, sharing some small personal details as a way to test a person's ability to be trusted, or simply taking time to get to know people slowly are all good approaches.

_____

_____

_____

Practicing gratitude in relationships can help keep your focus on the healthy, positive parts of those relationships while also helping you maintain a hopeful perspective when you're working through relationship challenges. Be intentional about infusing your relationships with gratitude on a regular basis. Some ways you might practice gratitude in your relationships include sending a quick text message highlighting something you appreciate about the other person, sending a handwritten letter or card describing the impact they've had on you, or simply telling people on a regular basis that you're thankful for what they bring to your life.

_____

_____

_____

## EXERCISE 6: MENDING FENCES

Isolation is an abuse tactic that many abusers use to control their victims. It's common for victims of abuse to become isolated from others. In addition to the ways that your abuser actively isolated you from others, you may have noticed that friends, family members, and other close connections pulled away while you were facing abuse because they didn't know how to help you.

In addition to the direct hurts that your abuser inflicted on you, there may also be lingering hurt feelings in other relationships in your life as a result of the abuse you faced. On the following lines, identify at least three people with whom you might like to reconnect or mend a hurt relationship. Then, for each person you identify, list at least two steps you could take to open the door to rebuilding that relationship.

Person #1: _____

Relationship rebuilding step #1: _____

Relationship rebuilding step #2: _____

Person #2: _____

Relationship rebuilding step #1: _____

Relationship rebuilding step #2: _____

Person #3: _____

Relationship rebuilding step #1: _____

Relationship rebuilding step #2: _____

What are some relationship patterns you've experienced in your past, including relationship patterns you saw in your family of origin, that you don't want to repeat? What are some steps you can take to break out of these patterns?

_____

_____

## EXERCISE 7: MAKING NEW FRIENDS

It's hard to make new friends as an adult! You might feel a little embarrassed to admit it if you're finding it difficult to make friends in adulthood, but know that this is a very common experience. Making new friends can be even more challenging for survivors of abuse, especially if you still have lingering trust issues or lack self-confidence because of how your abuser treated you.

In this exercise, you'll brainstorm ideas for how you might expand your friendship network and then list those ideas below. Your list might include places or groups where you could meet people, ways you can make new connections, and opportunities to grow current acquaintances into closer friends. Be patient as you begin to put these ideas into practice, and keep in mind that friendships can take a long time to build. Try to enjoy the process and the opportunities to connect with new people, even if close relationships don't develop right away.

_____

_____

_____

_____

Especially during conflict, people have a tendency to focus on what they would like the other person to change. There's an important place for this in relationships, but it's also helpful to apply intentional self-reflection. Consider your own thoughts, behaviors, and expectations and how they're playing out in your relationships. Be mindful of your thoughts and feelings, especially in tense situations. Reflect on changes that you could make that might help your relationships change in a positive direction. Healthy relationships are a two-way street, but we can help improve the overall quality of our relationships by working on our own capacity and skills so we bring our best selves to the important relationships in our lives.

---

---

---

## Healthy Relationships Take Work and Intentional Effort

When you don't put in the work, your relationships can falter from neglect. However, healthy relationships shouldn't feel like hard labor! Find the right balance among work, comfort, enjoyment, and growth in your relationships. Over time, make sure that you and the people close to you are putting in relatively equivalent amounts of effort. When it comes to healthy relationships that stand the test of time, each person can contribute to the quality of the connection by working to support and nurture the relationship.

EXERCISE 8: HEALTHY CONFLICT

Did you know that conflict is an important part of healthy relationships? It's natural and expected that different people will bring different ideas and perspectives to relationships, and healthy conflict management skills can help people navigate these differences.

Of course, facing verbal abuse can warp your perspective because conflict with an abuser is often very unhealthy, and even unsafe. As you move forward in your abuse recovery process, work toward building and practicing healthy conflict resolution skills. In this exercise, check the appropriate box to rate yourself in terms of how effective you are in each of the conflict management skills listed below. Once you've identified your strengths and weaknesses, map out a plan to build stronger skills in the areas where you are currently weak.

| Conflict Management Skill | Not at all effective | Somewhat effective | Very effective |
|---|---|---|---|
| Staying calm during stressful, high-conflict situations | | | |
| Communicating your perspective without attacking the other person | | | |
| Listening calmly to try to understand the other person's perspective | | | |
| Working toward a mutually agreeable compromise or win-win solution | | | |
| Thinking creatively about solutions to conflict situations | | | |
| Apologizing if you say or do hurtful things during conflict situations | | | |
| Reconnecting in a healthy way following conflict | | | |

What are your favorite things about your closest relationships? In what ways do these relationships add joy and meaning to your life?

_____

## EXERCISE 9: OVERCOMING FEAR THAT OTHER PEOPLE WON'T LIKE YOU

Facing abuse can lead survivors to become especially sensitive about being liked by others. If your abuser tried to make you feel like an unlikable person, you may feel insecure about whether others will like you, even long after you're free from the abuse.

If you want to build healthy, authentic relationships with others, it's natural that some people may not like you when they get to know the real you. Likewise, you probably won't like everyone you get to know, either. Accepting that not everyone is meant to be part of your close inner circle can help you come nearer to finding the right people to be part of that group. To help you explore any potential underlying fears that others won't like you, reflect on the questions below.

To what extent do you experience fears that other people won't like you? How, if at all, were these fears exacerbated by your experiences with verbal abuse?

_____

_____

_____

How do any underlying fears about not being liked influence how you show up in relationships? How do these fears factor into your willingness to be authentic with others?

_____

_____

_____

What are some steps you could take to support yourself in moving beyond these fears so that you can become more free to be yourself in relationships?

_____

_____

_____

The best way to have good friends is to be a good friend to others. In this exercise, identify at least five current friends—even if you're not very close to them—and write down at least one specific way that you could be a good friend to each person in the next month.

Friend #1: _____

Friend #2: _____

Friend #3: _____

Friend #4: _____

Friend #5: _____

# CONCLUSION

Relationships can be a challenging part of life for people who have faced the hurt of abuse within important relationships in their lives. Regardless of any past relational hurts you have faced, you are worthy of healthy, respectful, and positive relationships in all areas of your life. In this chapter, we've explored topics and skills that can help you enhance your relationships, both during your abuse recovery process and throughout your life.

We've also highlighted the importance of intentionality when it comes to building and maintaining healthy relationships. As we head into the final chapter of this workbook, we'll bring this same level of intentionality to another exciting—and sometimes challenging—aspect of the long-term, ongoing work of abuse recovery: developing and pursuing dreams for your future.

## CHAPTER 7

# DREAMING FOR YOUR FUTURE

You've made it this far along in the *Verbal Abuse Recovery Workbook,* and you've likely come a long way in your abuse recovery process. It may seem as though you still have a lot more work and time ahead of you before you'll feel that this process is complete.

Healing and recovering from verbal abuse are ongoing processes. Some people eventually do feel that they have fully and completely healed, whereas other people feel as though healing will be a lifelong process. There truly is no right or wrong "end point" to abuse recovery. What is most important is that you feel good about where you're heading.

In this final chapter of the workbook, we'll look ahead toward the long-term, ongoing journey of recovery, while also working toward building an inspiring, positive outlook toward your future.

## Recovery Story: Tell Your Story

Before we delve into this chapter's exercises, let's take a moment to reflect on how far you've come in your abuse recovery process. Pause for a few moments to think back on what you consider the starting point of this process—it might be the moment you decided to end your relationship with your former abuser, the time when the relationship actually ended, a later point when you decided to get intentional about healing, or even when you first thought about going through this workbook.

Using whichever starting point makes the most sense to you, reflect on all the ways you have grown and healed already. Your progress may feel slow, fast, steady, or inconsistent. Whether you feel that you've come a little or a long way, honor the progress you have made, and consider what you can learn about the steps you've taken so far to continue your forward momentum.

The abuse recovery journey can be a long, uncertain one. Unlike some other goals you may pursue in life—such as paying off debt or running a race—recovering from abuse doesn't necessarily have a clear end point. Some survivors will eventually feel completely healed. Others find that recovering from abuse is a lifelong process, although one that usually becomes easier over time.

In the space below, reflect on what you imagine the "end" of your own abuse recovery process might look like. Do you anticipate that one day you'll feel that this process is complete, or do you sense that it might be a lifelong journey? Regardless of whether you anticipate a clear end point, how will you know that your healing journey has been effective?

_____

_____

_____

_____

_____

_____

_____

_____

_____

_____

_____

_____

_____

_____

_____

_____

_____

A **vision board** offers a creative, tangible way to visualize what you hope to manifest in your life in the future. A vision board can be created in many ways, such as by creating a collage with magazine clippings or drawing and writing words on a piece of poster paper. You can look online for all sorts of ideas and inspiration. In this exercise, we'll focus on creating a vision board using a piece of paper (preferably larger poster board) and words and images cut from magazines as the primary materials.

This exercise involves building your supply list and plans to create a vision board that will support you on your healing journey. This vision board might be specific to what you hope for your healing specifically, or it may be a more general vision board for your life. Once you have your plans detailed, schedule some time on your calendar to start creating!

Supplies needed (add others you'd like to use in the lines below):

- Poster paper or other sturdy paper/cardboard
- Old magazines (your local library may have some you could take for free)
- Glue
- Scissors
- Other craft items to personalize your board (e.g., stickers, markers, paint, glitter)

    - _____

    - _____

    - _____

    - _____

Plans:

- Would I prefer to create my vision board alone, with one or more friends, or in some other setting?

    _____

    _____

- What time can I schedule to work on my vision board? (A window of two to three hours is recommended.)

    _____

    _____

- What inspirational music could I listen to? Or would I prefer to create my board in silence?

  _____

  _____

- What other steps can I take to make this vision board experience as comfortable and meaningful as possible? (Examples are buying snacks to enjoy while creating the board or planning to share the board with a trusted friend, family member, or professional once it is complete.)

  _____

  _____

- Where can I display my finished board to continue to motivate and inspire me?

  _____

  _____

## PROMPT 1: ANTICIPATING FUTURE BARRIERS

What are some potential barriers to your future progress along your abuse recovery journey? Examples may be procrastination, busyness, and feeling overwhelmed by the demands of day-to-day life. Once you've identified the barriers that are most relevant to you, how can you anticipate them and be proactive about managing them so they don't hinder your healing?

_____

_____

_____

_____

_____

_____

_____

_____

_____

## EXERCISE 3: PREPARING FOR SETBACKS

Progress along the journey of recovering from abuse usually isn't linear. You may feel like you take two steps forward, then one step back, then three steps forward, then two more steps back. Even though apparent setbacks can feel disheartening, try to stay focused on the positive progress you're making—as well as on learning and growing—whenever you face setbacks. If you're taking more steps forward than backward, you're still gaining ground!

Setbacks are part of any growth process in life. Below, list at least five reminders you can give yourself to help you stay motivated and positive, even when you face minor or major setbacks during your abuse recovery process.

*Example: Setbacks are disappointing, but they are a sign that I am making progress.*

1. _____

2. _____

3. _____

4. _____

5. _____

## PRACTICE 1: CREATE YOUR OWN HEALING EXERCISES

We've covered a lot of ideas for exercises and activities throughout this workbook. Some of these exercises likely resonated with you more than others. As you move forward beyond this book, consider how you can start to develop some self-created healing exercises and personalized homework that you assign yourself.

Trust your instincts, and consider the steps you could take to move forward further in your healing journey. Identify activities that you could work through to foster new opportunities for healing that are especially meaningful and personalized to your needs and experiences. There is value in trusting experts, books, and professionals along your healing process, but also listen to your own inner wisdom to identify steps you could take to keep moving forward.

_____

_____

_____

Each of us has an ongoing inner dialogue. Negative self-talk can hinder our personal growth. Be intentional about correcting negative self-talk patterns and replacing them with more positive, healing-oriented ones. In this exercise, practice replacing a negative self-talk statement with a more positive one, and repeat this process as you identify other negative self-talk patterns in your mind.

First, identify the negative self-talk statement or pattern. Do you repeat statements or patterns of statements in your mind that contribute to your feeling down or worse about yourself? If so, what are these statements?

_____

_____

_____

Next, critically examine how these self-talk patterns are impacting your life. What are some of the consequences of these patterns on your mental, emotional, and relational health?

_____

_____

_____

Finally, identify more accurate, positive self-talk patterns that you can repeat and practice reinforcing to help you overcome the negative self-talk patterns you identified above. Below, write at least three statements reflecting these more healing-oriented self-talk strategies.

1. _____

2. _____

3. _____

### PROMPT 2: DREAM BIG!

What is one big dream you have for your life? How, if at all, has surviving abuse helped increase your motivation for making this dream a reality?

_____

What can you do when your motivation starts to wane during your abuse recovery process? Staying motivated over the long term can be a challenge, especially when you face obstacles or are frustrated that progress is taking longer than you'd like. In this exercise, identify at least 10 "motivation boosters," or ideas for ways that you can reset your motivation if it begins to fade. These may include inspirational quotes, people who can encourage you, and resources you can consult to refresh your knowledge of the verbal abuse recovery process.

1. _____

2. _____

3. _____

4. _____

5. _____

6. _____

7. _____

8. _____

9. _____

10. _____

## Your Journey Is Your Own

Abuse recovery is a journey, not a one-time event. Your journey is your own. Don't feel as though you have to follow anyone else's timeline or process. Empower yourself along this journey to make decisions that are right for you. Continue to take small—and sometimes big—consistent steps forward. Eventually, you'll look back and be so proud of how far you've come.

Healing from verbal abuse usually involves a slow, steady process—it's more a marathon than a sprint, and it's important to find a pace and process that work for you. Taking a slow, steady approach will help you carve out moments and opportunities for healing that become a regular part of your daily and weekly schedule.

That said, you can add "healing accelerators" to your recovery process if you wish. Examples include intensive experiences, such as a retreat for survivors of abuse, personal growth workshops, or a solitary healing and meditation retreat.

Does this idea of "healing accelerators" appeal to you? How helpful might this approach be for your personal abuse recovery process?

_____

_____

_____

_____

If you find value in the concept of healing accelerators, what are some ideas that you might consider incorporating into your recovery journey?

_____

_____

_____

_____

### PROMPT 3: OVERCOMING A FEAR OF SUCCESS

What fears arise when you think about achieving your wildest dreams? Are you afraid they would take you away from some of the comforts in your life (e.g., relationships, habits)? What are some ways you could work toward overcoming any fear of success?

_____

_____

_____

Did you bury any big dreams or visions for your life as a result of the abuse you faced? Finish the sentence prompts below to help uncover these dreams or visions. Might you want to rebuild and expand on these buried dreams in the future?

When I was a child, I dreamed my life would be like . . .

_____

_____

_____

Before I faced verbal abuse, other dreams or hopes that I had for my future included . . .

_____

_____

_____

The abuse I faced impacted my ability to dream in the following ways:

_____

_____

_____

Dreams I'd like to revisit as I continue to move forward in my healing journey include . . .

_____

_____

_____

Some steps I can take to make time to explore these dreams include . . .

_____

_____

_____

You've probably heard the saying that life begins at the end of your comfort zone. Most of us don't love being uncomfortable and would prefer to feel safe and relaxed. But sometimes discomfort is a requirement for progress in life. Learn to embrace and appreciate discomfort when it serves as a catalyst for personal growth. Remind yourself when you face discomfort that it may not feel good, but it just might be good for you and your long-term progress. Develop a mantra or statement to repeat when you're intimidated by uncomfortable feelings or experiences, or when you're feeling that you'd prefer to avoid discomfort.

_____

_____

_____

_____

_____

_____

_____

_____

_____

_____

_____

During hard times, it can be difficult to experience joy and positivity. As we've discussed throughout this workbook, it's important to honor and process your emotions in a healthy, intentional way. Finding joy during difficult times does not mean glossing over or denying your pain; instead, it involves giving yourself permission to experience some joy and happiness, even if some aspects of your life are far from perfect.

The abuse recovery process is lengthy and difficult. You don't have to postpone all feelings of joy and positivity until that process is complete. You're worthy of experiencing joy and happiness, even if this happens only for brief moments at a time right now. Take time to reflect on the sources of joy that you can experience now. What are some ways you can give yourself opportunities to experience this joy, even during difficult times?

_____

_____

_____

_____

## PROMPT 4: HELPING OTHERS

Do you have a desire to help others who have faced similar abuse? It's okay if you don't! However, many survivors of abuse do aspire to help others who have had similar challenges. If you have a desire to help others, be intentional about this. Helping others can be a wonderful way to transform your experiences into a sense of meaning and purpose. Write some ideas for ways you could help others who have had similar abuse experiences or other related challenges in life. What steps could you take to put these ideas into action?

_____

_____

_____

_____

Facing abuse—and then the abuse recovery process—often leads survivors to some big-picture, existential questions. Examples of these questions are:

- What is the meaning of life?
- What is the purpose of suffering?
- Why did I have to go through this pain?

What are some of the existential questions that your own experiences with abuse and abuse recovery have brought up for you? How have your abuse and recovery experiences led you to new spiritual or existential insights that can help you further your growth?

_____

_____

_____

_____

## Remind Yourself of Your Worth

You are worthy of a positive future. Going through abuse can make you feel that you're not valued and worthy of respect, and those feelings can linger long after you're free from the abuse. Sometimes self-doubts can creep in and lead you to question your abilities or the chance for a brighter future. Continue to remind yourself of your worth. Surround yourself with others who will lift you up and let you know that you're worthy of hope for a peace-filled today and a positive, fulfilling future.

As we come to the end of this workbook, take some time to reflect on what you've learned and how you've grown as you've completed the exercises and activities. Complete the following sentence prompts to aid in this reflection.

Some insights I've gained about myself through this workbook include . . .

_____

_____

_____

Some areas in which I hope to continue to grow are . . .

_____

_____

_____

I was most surprised to learn . . .

_____

_____

_____

Recovering from abuse involves . . .

_____

_____

_____

I appreciate the work I've done because . . .

_____

_____

_____

## Recovery Story: The Future You

At the start of this chapter, I invited you to reflect on how far you've come already. Now, as we're reaching the end of the chapter and the workbook, take time to reflect in the other direction: the future. Envision what your future has in store for you, including possible challenges you'll face, but focus more attention on the positive experiences and relationships that you hope will come your way. Give yourself time to reflect on your hopes, fears, and dreams. As you look ahead, keep in mind that your life may not fully match your ideal vision of your future just yet, but you're making progress and heading in a positive direction.

# CONCLUSION

You can overcome the hurts and pains of your past, including the verbal abuse you experienced. In this chapter, you explored some of your hopes and dreams for your future, taking a realistic view that some progress will come with challenges and setbacks. Continue to stay hopeful and intentional as you progress through the long-term processes and growth involved in recovering from past abuse. Wherever your journey takes you, know that you are worthy of healing, respect, and inner peace.

# A FINAL WORD

Congratulations for doing the difficult yet important work of completing the *Verbal Abuse Recovery Workbook*! As you've worked your way through this book, you've explored different phases of the recovery process, developed self-care strategies that work for you, focused on building healthy relationships, and committed to the ongoing work of healing from past verbal abuse.

Every survivor has a unique and different experience of recovering from abuse. At this point, you might be excited by how far you've come, or you may feel frustrated because you'd hoped to feel further along by now. Trust that your healing journey is unfolding in a way that's right for you, and continue to explore ways to continue making progress. This might include repeating some or all of the exercises that we covered, delving into other books and resources, or seeking professional help. See the Resources section for additional information that can help you learn more about verbal abuse and the abuse recovery process.

I wish you the best as you continue to recover and heal from verbal abuse. I know from my personal and professional experiences that this is not an easy journey to be on. However, I encourage you to focus on the strengths and wisdom that you're gaining during this time and to know that your journey can continue until you decide that it's complete. Always embrace an underlying belief that you are worthy of kindness, respect, and self-love to guide you along the way.

# GLOSSARY

**gaslighting:** Occurs when an abuser plays mind games to try and confuse the victim or make them question their own reality, perceptions, and sanity

**manipulation:** A type of mind game in which someone is trying to trick or deceive someone else into doing something they want them to do or into getting them to take their side in a disagreement or debate

**name-calling:** Occurs when an abuser uses hurtful words toward the victim, such as by calling them dumb or cursing at them. Beyond these more obvious examples, however, name-calling can be more subtle, such as using nicknames or pet names that they know hurt the victim but that others may not immediately recognize as offensive.

**posttraumatic stress disorder (PTSD):** A diagnosable mental health disorder that describes a specific set of emotional and cognitive responses to a traumatic event or series of events. Some of the features of PTSD include anxiety, hypervigilance, avoidance of reminders of the traumatic event, and reexperiencing the event, such as through flashbacks or nightmares.

**safe relationships:** Relationships that are free from violence and abuse and provide a sense of physical and emotional safety and comfort

**SMART goals:** Goals that are Specific, Measurable, Action-Oriented, Realistic, and Time-Bound

**threatening:** May include physical harm, but also other potentially hurtful actions such as threatening harm to one's emotions, career or financial status, parenting situation, or status or reputation

**verbal abuse:** A pattern of using hurtful words and related actions to gain and maintain power and control over another person

**vision board:** A creative, tangible way to visualize what you hope to manifest in your life in the future. There are many ways to create a vision board, such as by doing a collage with magazine clippings or drawing and writing words on a piece of poster paper.

**withholding:** The absence of the level and type of positive words and associated behaviors that could reasonably be expected based on the nature of the relationship

# RESOURCES

## RESOURCES DEVELOPED BY THE AUTHOR AND HER COLLEAGUES:

The See the Triumph social media campaign for survivors of past intimate partner violence: SeeTheTriumph.org; Facebook and Pinterest: seethetriumph; Instagram: @triumphoverabuse

The Healthy Relationships Initiative, which offers resources and programs to promote happy, healthy, safe relationships of all kinds: HealthyRelationshipsInitiative.org; Facebook, Pinterest, and Instagram: @healthyrelationshipsinitiative

Christine Murray's website, which has resources related to violence and abuse, and updates on her work: ChristineMurray.info

The book *Triumph Over Abuse: Healing, Recovery, and Purpose after an Abusive Relationship* by Christine Murray, published in 2020 by Routledge Mental Health

## RESOURCES FOR SEEKING PROFESSIONAL HELP:

2-1-1 is a resource and referral service provided by United Way agencies: 211.org

Counselor Find from the National Board of Certified Counselors: NBCC.org/search/counselorfind

Find a Therapist from Psychology Today: PsychologyToday.com/us/therapists

The National Domestic Violence Hotline offers 24/7 support via phone, text, or chat: TheHotline.org

Therapist Locator from the American Association for Marriage and Family Therapy: TherapistLocator.net

# REFERENCES

Bancroft, Lundy. *Why Does He Do That? Inside the Minds of Angry and Controlling Men.* New York: Berkley Books, 2003.

Murray, Christine, E., Ratchneewan Ross, and Jennifer Cannon. "The Happy, Healthy, Safe Relationships Continuum: Conceptualizing a Spectrum of Relationship Quality to Guide Community-Based Healthy Relationship Promotion Programming." *The Family Journal* 29, no. 1 (2021): 50–59. doi.org/10.1177/1066480720960416.

# INDEX

# ACKNOWLEDGMENTS

I am grateful for the team at Callisto Media for the opportunity to write this workbook. In addition, I am thankful to the many survivors of past abuse who have shared their stories with me, whether through my research, teaching, counseling, community work, or friendships. Finally, I am grateful for the love and support of my friends and family, and especially my sons, Evan and Bryce. Thank you for always inspiring me to do my small part to contribute to building a more peaceful world.

# ABOUT THE AUTHOR

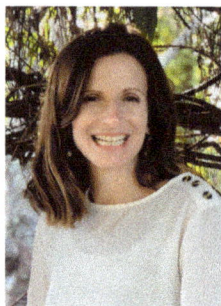

**Christine Murray, LCMHC, LMFT,** is the director of the Center for Youth, Family, and Community Partnerships at the University of North Carolina at Greensboro. Previously, she served for 14 years as a professor in the UNCG Department of Counseling and Educational Development, where she coordinated the Couple and Family Counseling track. Currently, she also directs the Healthy Relationships Initiative and is cofounder of the See the Triumph Campaign. To learn more about Christine's work, please visit ChristineMurray.info.

www.ingramcontent.com/pod-product-compliance
Lightning Source LLC
Chambersburg PA
CBHW050256090426

42734CB00022B/3478